The SIBO Cookbook for the Newly Diagnosed

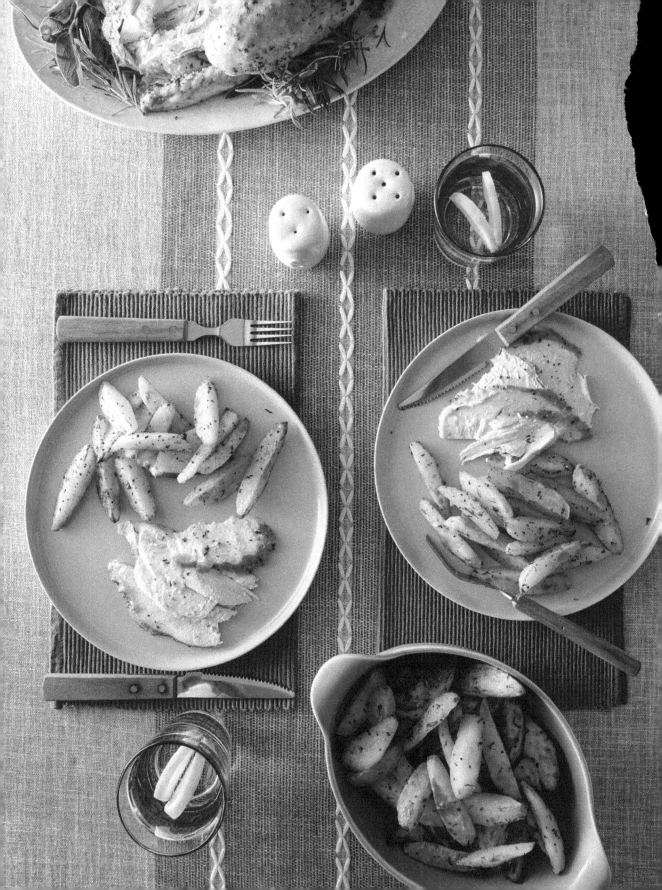

THE
SIBO
COOKBOOK
FOR THE
NEWLY DIAGNOSED

The Complete Guide to Relieving Symptoms and Preventing Recurrence

Kristy Regan, MScN

PHOTOGRAPHY BY DARREN MUIR

**ROCKRIDGE
PRESS**

For general information on our other products and services or to obtain technical support, please contact our Customer Care Department within the U.S. at (866) 744-2665, or outside the U.S. at (510) 253-0500.

Rockridge Press publishes its books in a variety of electronic and print formats. Some content that appears in print may not be available in electronic books, and vice versa.

Interior and Cover Designer: Joshua Moore
Photo Art Director/Art Manager: Sara Feinstein
Editor: Sean Newcott
Production Editor: Kurt Shulenberger
Photography © 2019 Darren Muir. Food styling by Yolanda Muir. Author photo courtesy of Emily V. Whellbarger.

ISBN: Print 978-1-64152-986-0 | eBook 978-1-64152-987-7
R0

To my dear husband, Gregg—
it's all so much more fun with you.

To my parents, Dad, Mom, Aira, and
Arthur—thank you for everything.

● ● ●

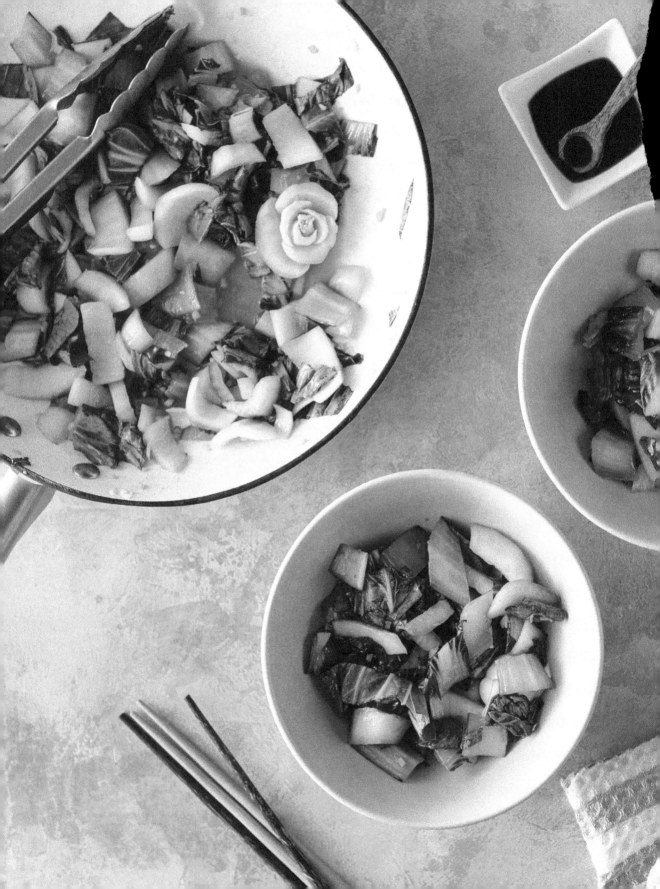

Contents

Foreword

THIS NEW COOKBOOK IS THE LATEST EXAMPLE OF Kristy Regan's user-friendly, well-informed, practical, creative, and well-written work. The clear, concise discussion of small-intestine bacterial overgrowth (SIBO) that leads into the healing recipes is the product of years of study, scholarly discussions, and symposia that she has not only attended but lectured at and even co-organized. She continues to be a great asset to physicians working in the field of functional gastroenterology.

I am a naturopathic gastroenterologist and over the last two decades have lectured about digestive health and disease. I supervise student doctors working with patients suffering from complex digestive conditions. I met Kristy about a decade ago when she was a student in the Master of Science in Nutrition program at the National University of Natural Medicine. She chose to attend one of my clinic rotations weekly for a year to help our patients with their diets. She was especially focused on diets for SIBO and related conditions. Since her graduation, I have called on her to help many of my patients with the ins and outs of diet, nutrition, cooking, and support.

Many of my patients have told me how helpful Kristy's first cookbook, *The SIBO Diet Plan*, has been. This new volume gives us more recipes to enjoy and additional resources to navigate the essential process of individualizing a diet for those newly diagnosed with SIBO. I especially appreciate that this cookbook includes recipe labels and nutritional labels. These list the various diets for which the recipe is appropriate and essential categories (dairy-free, gluten-free, nut-free, and vegetarian).

I work with many people dealing with SIBO. In addition to the pain and dysfunction they experience, they are frustrated with how their diet has been restricted by the condition. It is not uncommon to hear from patients that they have lost much of their interest in food and eating. When Kristy writes, "Reset your gut but enjoy your life," it is the hope that my patients are searching for. Kristy helps my patients keep their joy and passion for food, cooking, and a life well lived. I thank her for this gift.

The machine used to test breath samples for SIBO has been around since the 1970s. There have been descriptions of SIBO in almost every major textbook of medicine and pathology (it is also called "bacterial overgrowth syndrome" or "blind loop syndrome"). When Dr. Allison Siebecker and I started researching SIBO in 2009, these descriptions were very short and very little was known about mechanisms, details of diagnosis, treatment, or prevention.

Kristy has been working side by side with us during most of this long process. When we started this, we did not realize how important and huge SIBO research was and how large the field would become. More recently, many nutritionists have jumped on the bandwagon and have declared themselves "experts" in diet for SIBO. Kristy is the real thing.

Steven Sandberg-Lewis, ND, DHANP
Portland, Oregon, August 2019

Introduction

DID YOU KNOW THAT UP TO 84 PERCENT OF PEOPLE with irritable bowel syndrome (IBS) may actually have small-intestine bacterial overgrowth (SIBO)? Since IBS affects up to 45 million people in the U.S., that is over 37 million diagnosed and undiagnosed cases of SIBO. So even if you feel alone right now, the statistics say that you are, beyond a doubt, not in this by yourself. Having a community is important, especially when you have SIBO. Please know that many other people like you are seeking support, and there are many health professionals who care immeasurably and want to help you. I know it can be scary to have been diagnosed or suspect you have SIBO. This book is here to show you that it is possible to manage your SIBO and live a healthy, wonderful life filled with delicious food.

When I was diagnosed many years ago with SIBO, no one I knew had ever heard of it, including me. I always considered myself a healthy person, so to be in a state of chronic illness challenged who I knew myself to be in multiple ways. Looking back at my health journey, sometimes I did the right things, but sometimes I was the "what not to do" poster child. I saw a doctor a couple of times and then tried to make it on my own for about a year before deciding to find a new doctor. I fanatically adhered to a restrictive diet for a long time. I was always hungry from malabsorption, so I snacked throughout the day. I ate solid food the day after stopping an elemental diet (a fully liquid diet). I never saw a nutritionist or a mental health-care professional, both of whom I could have used.

It is not that I was careless, weak, or uninformed. There just was not a lot of information available at the time, and what was available was often conflicting. It was challenging to figure out why I was having specific symptoms. There were way too many diets, and no one could guarantee which one would work.

And yet, by working with my own body's cues, becoming highly edu-cated about SIBO, finding the right diet, understanding my underlying cause, and making lifestyle changes, I finally began to heal. Of course, I also had the help of some really amazing professionals without whom I could not have done it. Even though my road had a lot of twists and turns, I did get better. There is definitely hope for everyone.

For years now, I have been supporting people who are dealing with and healing from SIBO. I am so happy to be able to condense my understanding of nutrition, SIBO-friendly diets and recipes, and general SIBO knowledge into this book for you. I have made this information as straightforward and accessible as possible. What you are feeling is completely normal. It can be scary, frustrating, and sometimes painful living with SIBO, and managing it can seem confusing. This book is here to guide you and give you everything you need to know to go down the path into better health.

I won't lie; there is work ahead for you. It may involve changing your diet, learning to cook and thinking about cooking from a new vantage point, reviewing the role of stress in your everyday life, and rethinking how you interact with friends and family. There is a lot to learn about SIBO, but the great part is that it is here, easily readable, organized, and ready for you to begin.

You are not alone in this SIBO journey, and I am excited to be one of your advocates.

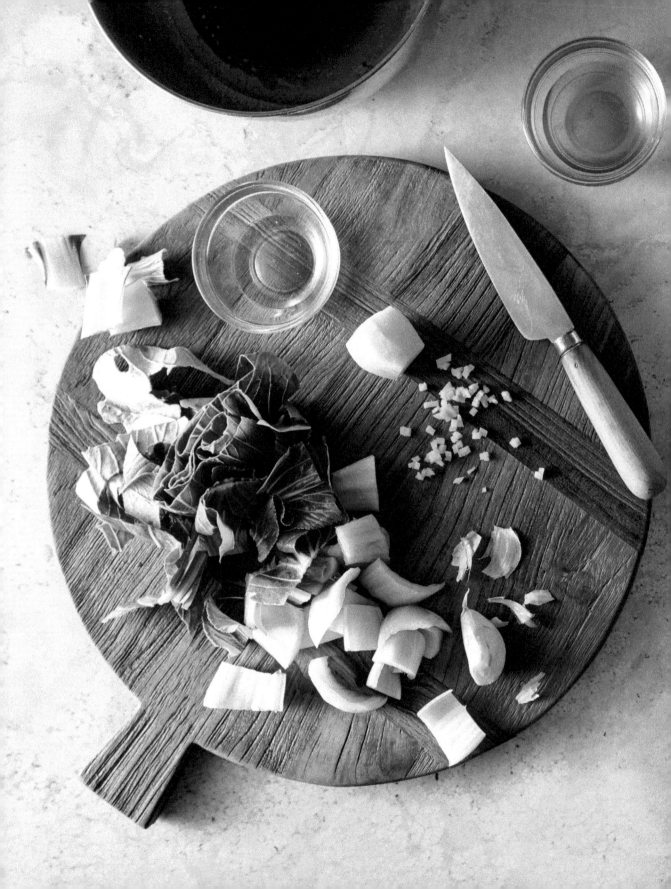

PART ONE

Small-Intestine Bacterial Overgrowth

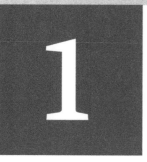

Understanding SIBO

THIS CHAPTER WILL SERVE AS A RESOURCE FOR understanding what SIBO (small-intestine bacterial overgrowth) is and how a healthy digestive system differs from one that is out of balance because of a bacterial overgrowth. Although SIBO research is still in its infancy, we are finding out more every day about how gut health is connected to our overall system health. As more scientists study and learn about SIBO, more and more people dealing with this issue are being officially diagnosed. If you have been misdiagnosed, told you could not be helped, or are just starting to realize you need support with your gastrointestinal issues, please know that your symptoms are valid and SIBO is a legitimate disorder. The information in this book will be an integral piece of your support system.

SIBO

SIBO is defined as an overgrowth of bacteria in the small intestine. When an overgrowth occurs, a variety of gastrointestinal symptoms may present themselves. Some people with SIBO won't go to a doctor at all because they are embarrassed by their symptoms, do not think it is that serious, or hope the symptoms will just go away on their own. For those who do see a doctor, SIBO is still largely undiagnosed, so people may be misdiagnosed with other gastrointestinal issues or told that they just have to live with their condition. As more research and studies are completed, the misdiagnoses will go down in number.

The Digestive System

Your digestive system, when functioning properly, is a marvel to behold. Its goal is to break down and absorb nutrients. The digestive system is made up of hollow organs such as the mouth, esophagus, stomach, small intestine, large intestine, and anus. They are hollow so that food and by-products can travel through them. The system's solid organs are the pancreas, liver, and gallbladder, and the supporting players are the nervous and circulatory systems, as well as gut bacteria.

Digestion really starts when you begin to think about or smell food. (That is why "fast food" is often thought of as unhelpful to the digestive system: There is not a lot of time between the initial thought of food and actually getting it.) When you cook, talk about, smell, serve, and enjoy your food in a relaxed state, your digestive system has more time to activate and is more likely and better able to process food well. I want to walk you through the technical process of healthy digestion to show you how everything in your body is supposed to work together to digest food properly.

The salivary glands produce saliva, which is made of water, electrolytes, and enzymes. When you take a bite of food, the saliva helps moisten and lubricate food as well as dissolve it. It also provides anti-bacterial protection. As the first part of the process of digestion, it is very important to chew your food mindfully and thoroughly to support the rest of the digestion process.

After you chew your food, it becomes a bolus, which is a chewed-up mass. Once you swallow the bolus, it enters the esophagus and your body takes over to perform the rest of digestion. The esophagus is signaled from your brain, and peristalsis begins. Peristalsis is a series of involuntary muscle contractions that take place in the esophagus, stomach, and intestines to move the bolus through the system.

The bolus enters the stomach, which contains hydrochloric acid and pepsin, our gastric juices. Peristalsis continues in the stomach, mixing food with the gastric juices. The food stays in the stomach for one to two hours, turning into a thick mixture called "chyme," and then it exits through the pyloric sphincter into the small intestine.

The small intestine is about 20 feet long. The duodenum is the first part of the small intestine. In the duodenum, the chyme mixes with liver bile to help break down fats, pancreatic juices (including the enzymes trypsinogen, elastase, and amylase), and intestinal juices that activate the enzymes. The chyme continues to be digested as it travels to the latter parts of the small intestine, the jejunum and ileum. The ileocecal valve is the valve between the small and large intestine. It is meant to be a one-way valve from the small to the large intestine, but if there is backflow, then it is possible for bacteria to pass from the large intestine back up into the small intestine.

The large intestine, also called the colon or large bowel, is about five feet in length and is wider than the small intestine. It absorbs water and minerals into the blood. Gut bacteria ferment the chyme and absorb any by-products of fermentation, such as vitamin B_{12}, vitamin K, thiamine, and riboflavin.

Any waste from the colon is passed to the rectum and is excreted via the anus.

THE IMPORTANCE OF THE SMALL INTESTINE

The main function of the small intestine is to absorb nutrients and minerals from the food we eat. The small intestine typically houses a small number of bacteria, especially compared to the large intestine, which is home to trillions of bacteria. The bacteria in the small intestine, however, have a major job to do; they protect against harmful bacteria and yeast as well as help absorb nutrients.

We have multiple protections against bacterial overgrowth. For one, the hydrochloric acid in the stomach kills bacteria in the food we consume. Bile and enzymes arrest bacterial growth, the immune system is set up to eradicate anything offending, and the ileocecal valve prevents backflow from the large intestine. Lastly, the migrating motor complex (MMC) performs a sweeping wave in the small intestine to move bacteria, cellular debris, and any indigestible food out of the small intestine.

Bacteria and Gut Health

When a bacterial overgrowth occurs in the small intestine, it is not necessarily from pathogenic (bad) bacteria. It is specifically a location issue since larger numbers of bacteria should be in the large intestine, not the small intestine. When a bacterial overgrowth accumulates in the small intestine, the bacteria may consume nutrients, such as B_{12} or iron, before they can be absorbed into your body. These bacteria can damage the lining of the small intestine, causing leaky gut syndrome. In the case of leaky gut, larger food particles can enter the bloodstream. If the immune system reacts to those particles, food intolerances or allergies can result. SIBO and leaky gut are often both present together, but they do not always occur concurrently.

SIBO also has an overall high recurrence rate. Addressing the underlying cause while also eradicating bacterial overgrowth is of the utmost importance. Damage to the MMC (the sweeper wave of the small intestine) is a common underlying cause, and if that is the case, it is imperative to support the MMC with prokinetics, which are medications to promote gastrointestinal motility and transit.

ANTIBIOTICS

Many health-care providers do not want to treat SIBO with herbal or pharmaceutical antibiotics since some patients have SIBO because of their overuse of antibiotics in the first place. Currently, however, it is the treatment that has the most studied advocacy. That said, doctors should still be careful with how and when antibiotics are administered. Some patients are prescribed rounds of antibiotics over and over again without a reevaluation of their full health picture. Wiping out one's microbiome can bring its own consequences and symptoms. Even someone who responded well to their SIBO treatments may see a negative change in their microbiome. In the aftermath of SIBO, most people will need to review the state of their large-intestine gut bacteria and build it back to a healthy condition over time.

SIBO RECURRENCE

Treatment may involve addressing multiple issues, not just SIBO. When the gut is damaged or if there is immune system dysfunction, it may make you more susceptible to parasites, yeast overgrowth, large-intestine dysbiosis, and a host of other issues. For people with SIBO, the journey to wellness can take time and focus, and it is incredibly important to have the right health team in place.

Some doctors who are not used to treating SIBO may recommend just one round of antibiotics without paying attention to the severity of the bacterial overgrowth. They may not retest for the presence of SIBO after a previous round of antibiotics to see how their patient responded to that treatment. Many times, a patient responds well to one protocol but not another, so it is important for both the doctor and the patient to follow up and not assume it will be a "one and done" situation. As the patient, you can request a follow-up SIBO test, even if the doctor doesn't necessarily feel that it is merited. In addition to being vigilant about your health, a course of action like a prokinetic after-treatment can make a huge difference in keeping your SIBO from recurring.

The Different Types of SIBO

Different types of SIBO are linked to different types of bacteria or archaea overgrowth. These types are often linked to particular symptoms, although each person is unique. The type of SIBO may also be treated with different herbal or pharmaceutical antibiotics, so it is important for you to understand which type of SIBO you have.

HYDROGEN-DOMINANT SIBO

Hydrogen (H_2) gas is produced by hydrogen-gas–producing bacterial overgrowths, making for hydrogen-dominant SIBO. People with hydrogen-dominant SIBO are typically more prone to diarrhea. In addition to diarrhea, people may have malabsorption of nutrients and will then be more prone to unwanted weight loss.

If you have ongoing diarrhea, your electrolytes need to stay balanced, so drinking a homemade electrolyte drink is often helpful. (See the recipe for Maple Ginger Electrolyte Drink on page 153.) For unwanted weight loss, it is important to eat healthy fat and carbohydrate combinations and to take in extra calories with beverages during meals when possible. In addition to regular meals, people may also benefit from an easily absorbable elemental diet drink, like the one from Integrative Therapeutics (see the Resources section on page 164 for more information). This will provide easily assimilated calories and nutrients in addition to your regular food intake.

METHANE-DOMINANT SIBO

Originally, methane-dominant SIBO was also thought to be caused by a bacterial overgrowth, but we now know that methane (CH_4) gas is caused by archaea, a single-celled organism. Nevertheless, it is still put into the overarching category of a bacterial overgrowth. Typical symptoms of methane-dominant SIBO may include bloating, constipation, and flatulence.

MIXED-TYPE SIBO

With mixed-type SIBO, both methane and hydrogen-related overgrowths are present and need to be addressed. If one type is more present, the symptoms may be more related to that type, or they may fluctuate over time. If methane is more dominant and goes down when a treatment protocol is administered, sometimes the hydrogen goes up because there are more free hydrogen molecules (H_2) from the breakup of methane molecules (CH_4).

For hydrogen-dominant, methane-dominant, and mixed-type SIBOs, the general dietary changes are often the same, although they should be tailored to an individual's tolerances and symptoms.

HYDROGEN-SULFIDE SIBO

At the time of the writing of this book, there is not yet a test for hydrogen sulfide (H_2S) SIBO, although Dr. Mark Pimentel of Cedars-Sinai Medical Center plans to release a new four-gas breath-test device that will test for hydrogen-sulfide SIBO in addition to the hydrogen- and methane-dominant types by the end of 2019. Currently, doctors diagnose hydrogen-sulfide SIBO from a flatline lactulose breath test and accompanying specific symptoms related to hydrogen-sulfide SIBO. A flatline test means that the readings for both hydrogen and methane gas tend to be in the low ranges throughout the test. It will also look like a flatline on the accompanying test graph.

Symptoms related to hydrogen-sulfide SIBO may include sulfuric- or rotten-egg–smelling gas, belching, bladder irritation, diarrhea (although some people may experience constipation instead or alternating symptoms), nausea, rashes, and body pain.

With hydrogen-sulfide SIBO, it can be helpful to adopt a low-sulfur diet for at least a week and see if it makes a difference in symptoms. If it does, that does not necessarily mean that a person will react to all foods high in sulfur, so it is helpful to test for them individually in the long run. In addition, some people maintain a low-FODMAP diet. (FODMAP stands for fermentable oligosaccharides, disaccharides, monosaccharides, and polyols—scientific terms for different groups of carbohydrates.) But one study shows that a low-FODMAP diet may not be helpful for hydrogen-sulfide SIBO.

With new information and research still becoming available, it is incredibly important to test foods to each individual's tolerance. See the Resources section (page 164) for more information on low-sulfur diets.

Common Causes of SIBO

SIBO is not typically a condition that shows up in isolation, which often makes finding the underlying cause of one's SIBO a confusing task. Even the definition of "underlying cause" can be bewildering. In the case of SIBO, an underlying cause is simply what was present or changed in the body to allow an overgrowth to occur. Underlying causes can be structural or functional. The most common underlying cause is dysfunction of the MMC. The MMC provides a cleansing sweep of the small intestine about every 90 minutes during periods of fasting. If the MMC is not functioning as it should, bacteria are not swept away properly, setting the stage for a bacterial overgrowth in the small intestine.

Structurally, altered anatomy is another common underlying cause of SIBO. This can include partial obstructions in the small intestine from tumors, adhesions, twists, kinks, or strictures. If it is not functioning correctly, the ileocecal valve can also play a role in the overgrowth. The ileocecal valve is supposed to be a one-way valve from the small to the large intestine, but if there are issues, it may create a back migration, allowing more bacteria into the small intestine.

RISK FACTORS

Risk factors are essentially the root of the underlying cause. Just having a risk factor does not necessarily mean you will automatically get SIBO, but it will put you at a higher risk. Many risk factors exist for SIBO, and people can have more than one. The most common one is food poisoning, which damages the interstitial cells of Cajal (ICC); these control the MMC. To add insult to injury, once you have had food poisoning, you become more sensitive to it and are more likely to react to and be affected by it again. Many people look back in their history and can remember when they had a serious bout of gastroenteritis while visiting another country, whereas others might remember something far less severe, such as a light stomach flu or even just a stomachache. But either of those could be food poisoning, which may damage the MMC.

Other risk factors that can damage the MMC include Parkinson's disease, Ehlers-Danlos syndrome, diabetes, hypothyroidism, scleroderma, opiate and antibiotic use, and general stress. Obstructions or adhesions can result from surgeries, injuries, appendicitis, cancer, or irritable bowel disease (IBD). Low stomach acid (hypochlorhydria) may also be an issue.

Hypochlorhydria might be present on its own, or it can be the result of taking proton-pump inhibitors (PPIs). Many people with gastroesophageal reflux disease (GERD) or other conditions are put on PPIs for extended periods of time, which lowers their stomach acid. Unfortunately, a 2015 study found that the long-term use of PPIs is correlated to SIBO and other possible issues, including risk of pneumonia, fractures, vitamin B_{12} deficiency, chronic kidney disease, dementia, hypomagnesemia, and *Clostridium difficile* diarrhea.

In my practice, I notice that many of my clients have a history of low-level gastrointestinal symptoms with one or more structural or functional issues and risk factors over time, followed by a period of stress and at some later point a diagnosis of SIBO. This certainly will not be the case for everyone, but it is interesting to review our medical history to see what might have contributed to our current state of health.

COMPLICATIONS

When SIBO is left untreated, multiple issues can occur. The overgrowth of bacteria consumes nutrients like iron and vitamin B_{12}, possibly leading to anemia or low ferritin. The overgrowth results in deconjugated bile, which decreases fat absorption and possibly leads to vitamin A, E, D, and K deficiencies and fatty stools (steatorrhea). If the small intestine is damaged, larger food particles may enter the bloodstream. If there is an immune response, food allergies or intolerances can develop. Bacteria excretions may also lead to neurological issues.

This list does not include all the complications, but it reviews the most common ones. Speak with your doctor about any new issues, and if health-care providers are reviewing your blood work, it is important for them to know if you have been diagnosed with or suspect you have SIBO.

ASSOCIATED ISSUES

Many associated conditions or issues may exist in conjunction with SIBO, as well as be the cause or effect of SIBO. Some common ones include aging, anemia, anxiety, brain fog, celiac disease, chronic fatigue syndrome, chronic functional bloating, Crohn's disease, depression, Ehlers-Danlos syndrome, fibromyalgia, food poisoning, fructose malabsorption, GERD, *H. pylori* infection, hypochlorhydria, hypothyroidism, irritable bowel syndrome (IBS), leaky gut, malabsorption, malnutrition, mast cell activation syndrome (MCAS), parasites, Parkinson's disease, rheumatoid arthritis, rosacea, surgery, ulcerative colitis, and vitamin deficiencies.

A 2003 study found that up to 84 percent of people diagnosed with IBS also had SIBO. It is estimated that IBS affects between 24 million and 45 million people in the United States alone and 10 to 15 percent of the worldwide population. Other than a low-FODMAP diet to mitigate symptoms, there has not been a direct way to address IBS. But if you previously thought you had IBS or were diagnosed, it is a good time to see if you also have SIBO.

SIBO Knowledge Is Wellness Power

Learning about SIBO can be overwhelming, and you might be feeling frustrated and exhausted, but with the straightforward, scientific information in this first chapter, you should have a thorough understanding of healthy digestion, the different types of SIBO, and how SIBO affects your body. The journey to a healthier state may have several twists and turns, but you are learning about your well-being and what you need to move toward it. By reading this book, you are igniting your self-advocacy and starting to address your SIBO. There is a lot of power in that first step.

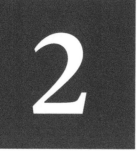

2

SIBO Symptoms

THIS CHAPTER WILL COVER THE DIFFERENT SYMPTOMS of SIBO and how they manifest. Unfortunately, many people can start to feel disconnected from or even betrayed by their bodies because of their SIBO symptoms. Sometimes SIBO patients encounter health-care providers who do not believe that their symptoms or SIBO itself is real, but SIBO *is* real, and our bodies are doing their absolute best to speak to us when we are eating something that is not supportive.

For those newly diagnosed with SIBO, it can be helpful to keep a journal that records daily food intake, symptoms, and bowel movements. This way, with the help of a SIBO-literate doctor, nutritionist, or other health-care provider, you can ascertain patterns and information over time and begin to translate what your body is telling you. Your most important job is to be a steadfast ally to your body and an unwavering advocate for yourself.

SIBO Symptoms: What You Feel Is Real

The first thing to remember is that SIBO symptoms are not just your imagination. They tend to be cyclic or ongoing rather than a short-term or one-time symptom that people may experience if they ate something too rich, if they ate too much, or if something did not agree with them.

For people with SIBO, high-fiber foods often make their symptoms worse because a bacterial overgrowth consumes fermentable foods and releases gases. People with SIBO may notice that their symptoms increased after a bout of food poisoning or stomach flu, after surgery, or after the use of proton-pump inhibitors (PPIs), opiates, or frequent antibiotics.

There are too many SIBO symptoms to list them all, but here are some of the more common ones. Possible short-term symptom-mitigation solutions are offered for some symptoms, but please remember that this should not be construed as or used in place of professional medical advice. Always refer to your doctor or health-care provider before making changes.

Diarrhea: Diarrhea tends to be linked to hydrogen-dominant SIBO, but it may also be seen in hydrogen-sulfide SIBO and mixed-type SIBO. Diarrhea may range from soft stools with clear-cut, ragged, or fuzzy edges to stools that partially or completely dissipate once hitting the toilet water to liquid stools with no solid pieces.

▶ To help mitigate system imbalances from diarrhea, it is important to stay hydrated and replenish electrolytes with an electrolyte-rich drink (such as the Maple Ginger Electrolyte Drink—see page 153). Some people experience reduced symptoms when they introduce a probiotic (*Saccharomyces boulardii* has been found in studies to be efficacious for those with diarrhea). For some, returning to a very basic diet (meat, white potato or white rice as tolerated, and one or two tolerated vegetables) for one to three days may be helpful.

Constipation: Constipation is typically associated with methane-dominant SIBO, although some people with hydrogen-dominant or mixed-type SIBOs experience both constipation and diarrhea. Those with constipation may have fewer bowel movements as well as harder ones that are more challenging to pass. Eating more fiber often results in more symptoms rather than decreased constipation.

▶ To ease constipation, make sure to include healthy fats in your diet. You can take fish oil capsules in the dosage recommended on the bottle or fish oil liquid. With the liquid, start with one teaspoon a day and move up to one tablespoon daily. When I take the liquid, I always chase it with water to avoid the fishy taste. For some people, castor-oil packs on the stomach can relieve both constipation and bloating. Castor-oil-pack kits are available online, or you can easily make your own (see the Resources section on page 164 for more information). Epsom salt baths are relaxing and have a gentle laxative effect. Magnesium can also be helpful for constipation; start with a lower dose and work up to a higher one as needed.

Flatulence and Belching: When gases are released from a bacterial overgrowth, the body often liberates that gas with flatulence or belching. Of course, everyone experiences some flatulence or belching normally, but the amount associated with SIBO feels markedly different for most people, or they feel like they have always had more than other people. In these cases, they may have had overgrowths for an ongoing period.

▶ Iberogast, an herbal formula originally created in Europe, can be useful for a variety of conditions, including gas and belching. Try 20 drops in ⅛ cup of warm water at each meal or when you are experiencing symptoms. Using a digestive enzyme with meals can also support digestion and lessen flatulence or belching.

Bloating, Cramping, or Abdominal and Bowel Pain: When gases are trapped and not released, bloating often occurs. This can create abdominal distention, an uncomfortable feeling of fullness, or pain. Many people with SIBO start the day with a little or some bloating, and it increases throughout the day. Some women are even mistaken for looking pregnant due to the amount of bloating. The trapped gas can also cause abdominal or bowel pain or cramping, which may also be due to bowel irritation.

▶ Castor-oil-pack kits can also ease bloating and abdominal pain, as can the Iberogast we discussed for flatulence and belching. Using a digestive enzyme with meals can support digestion and may lessen the bloating or cramping in conjunction with meals. A prokinetic supplement such as Motility Activator may also be helpful.

Acid Reflux or GERD: Acid reflux or GERD (gastroesophageal reflux disease) symptoms can include chest pain, regurgitation of food, difficulty swallowing, heartburn (a burning sensation in the chest, typically after eating), or stomach acid flowing back into the esophagus (the tube connecting the stomach and the mouth). This affects some people with SIBO and may be caused by a hiatal hernia. In the case of a hiatal hernia, the stomach bulges up into the diaphragm, where normally the esophagus would attach to the stomach.

▶ Taking a digestive enzyme with meals may prevent or lessen the reflux associated with eating. Taking 20 drops of Iberogast with meals may also be helpful, as well as herbal bitters. One teaspoon of apple cider vinegar mixed into one cup of water before meals may also support digestion and lessen reflux. And there are both over-the-counter and prescription medications for acid reflux and heartburn.

Food Sensitivities: Food intolerances can occur when one has SIBO and increased symptoms from eating foods higher in FODMAP, fiber, starch, or resistant starch. Food sensitivities may occur if someone has leaky gut syndrome, and intestinal permeability can in turn result in more food sensitivities.

▶ Food sensitivities change over time, but taking a digestive enzyme with meals and finding a diet that lessens symptoms may be the most supportive change. To identify specific sensitivities, you can try an elimination diet and see if your symptoms lessen.

Fatigue: People with SIBO often experience fatigue for a variety of reasons. Weakness and fatigue are the typical symptoms of a vitamin B_{12} deficiency. Many people with SIBO also experience disturbed sleep because of blood sugar or other issues and therefore have daytime fatigue. Adrenal issues may also come into play in relation to SIBO. It is important to speak with your doctor to specifically address the reason for fatigue.

NOT ALL SIBO SYMPTOMS ARE THE SAME

Some doctors or other health-care providers may assume that if your SIBO symptoms are not typical ones, then you do not have SIBO and there is no reason to test for it. However, your symptoms are real, and even if they do not fall perfectly into the typical symptom spectrum, it is still possible that you have it. Here are some SIBO symptoms to look out for that are less typical but may still be present.

Weight Loss: Weight loss may be seen in more severe cases of SIBO where malabsorption is present. This is more typical of hydrogen-dominant SIBO. If you are eating the same amount of food but you always feel hungry and are losing weight, malabsorption may be a serious issue. People also tend to lose weight if they adopt a restrictive SIBO diet that significantly changes their caloric intake. They may not know what to eat, so they just end up eating less overall. Even if weight loss may seem desirable to some people, it is important to keep an eye on changes and not create disordered eating patterns.

▶ For those who are underweight or are losing weight too quickly, it is important to eat fat and carbohydrate combinations when possible and drink higher-calorie beverages during meals. Adding an elemental diet formula (like the one from Integrative Therapeutics) as a meal supplement (not a replacement) may also support weight retention, as it is easy to absorb. This formula is typically used when doing the elemental diet as a treatment, but it can also serve as a dietary supplement to add more calories.

Weight Gain: Weight gain is more common with methane-dominant SIBO and for those who tend to be more constipated. Weight gain may also be a consequence of hormonal changes or thyroid issues in conjunction with SIBO. These possibilities should be reviewed with your doctor.

▶ To address weight gain, see your doctor first to check if the change is from an underlying medical issue.

Nausea: Nausea may be due to delayed gastric emptying, fat malabsorption, or histamine intolerance. It can be helpful to use a supplement such as Motility Activator from Integrative Therapeutics or Iberogast to support gastric emptying and gastrointestinal transport.

▶ Ginger tea, tinctures, or supplements can ease nausea. Twenty drops of Iberogast in water with food may also reduce nausea.

Skin Issues: SIBO has been linked to a plethora of skin issues, including acne, rosacea, and skin inflammation. A 2008 study showed that the eradication of SIBO was connected with a regression of rosacea. Those with histamine intolerance may experience skin issues such as itching, swelling, or hives.

▶ For skin issues, it may be helpful to try a low-histamine diet to see if it lessens skin symptoms.

TRACKING YOUR SIBO SYMPTOMS

It can be extremely helpful to track your SIBO symptoms to see how they change and hopefully get better over time. Symptoms can be noted specifically with a number between 1 and 10 to gauge the level of each symptom. Instead of recording "stomach pain," you might write, "Persistent pressure on the upper left side of stomach after eating at a level of 5." When I had SIBO, I kept a sheet noting each symptom, how it was being addressed, and whether that was using a SIBO treatment, supplements, or other wellness practices. Each week, I added an update so I could review it with my doctor. This was really useful because it allowed me to specifically check in on symptoms that I may have forgotten about because they were getting better or were not the worst symptoms that week. If a specific symptom was worse, I could review my food diary to see if there might be a correlation with what I was eating, my stress level, how busy I was, or my sleep patterns.

Tracking your symptoms is important, but it should not be your only focus. Russell Delman, a wise teacher of mine, once told me that feeling whole leads to healing rather than healing leading to feeling whole. With SIBO and other chronic and life-changing medical conditions, we often wait for the condition to go away so we can feel whole again—the way we imagine we used to feel. But if we cannot find ways to feel whole with SIBO, it is likely there may always be some sort of real or imagined obstacle in our path to feeling whole.

Not that feeling whole while being sick is easy—it is quite the opposite. It is hard work, but it is certainly a worthwhile endeavor with many benefits. How one goes about doing that can be very specific to each individual, but I have found that practices such as meditation, gratitude, and mind-body integration especially resonate with and support me.

SIBO IS NOT CONTAGIOUS

SIBO is not contagious, nor is it an infection. It is simply an overgrowth of bacteria in the wrong place—the small intestine. Even though it is not contagious, people still tend to feel ashamed to talk about symptoms like diarrhea, bloating, constipation, and other IBS-related symptoms. Many of my clients, when they start to describe their symptoms, apologize for how specific they are being. I tell them that not only is it important to be specific but it is also something we will talk about a lot. This can be very freeing for people, especially when they develop a community of health-care providers and even friends with whom they feel comfortable sharing these details. It is important to have this because healthy bowel function is such an integral part of health, and our health is something worthy of talking about, learning about, and fighting for.

The Link between Mental Health and a Healthy Gut

Many people with diagnosed SIBO or who are experiencing SIBO symptoms encounter neurological symptoms or mood changes. Before my diagnosis, I was already a "worrier" and prone to low-level anxiety. But things definitely changed for me when I was at my sickest with SIBO. I isolated myself more and did not want to go out as much as I normally did. I was also highly emotional, quick to cry, extremely anxious, and constantly overwhelmed. At the time, I was enrolled in a rigorous academic program but learning and retaining information was very challenging. These changes I experienced have been echoed in studies on mice, in which their emotional behavior patterns shifted when their microbiomes were purposely and negatively changed.

As I began to heal over time, these symptoms eased, but my anxiety was the last to change. Although I am still a sensitive person who tends to be a slightly anxious overthinker, I no longer feel consistently overwhelmed. I have returned to what I know to be my neutral point. My experience seems fairly consistent with those of my clients; all of them have experienced some emotional distress or changes as a result of having SIBO. If you are feeling anxiety or other emotional sensitivity while going through and trying to diagnose and heal your SIBO, know that you are not alone in this.

The gut-brain axis is something commonly discussed in scientific circles and even the mainstream media these days. The gut-brain axis is bidirectional, meaning that changes in the gut bacteria affect the brain and that brain injuries or alteration can affect gut bacteria.

We often hear about stress in association with SIBO. Sometimes it is part of the cause, a symptom of SIBO, or the result of drastically changing your life while you are dealing with the condition. With all the effort one has to make—planning, cooking, research, health-care visits, reimagining social schedules and eating out, and so on—SIBO can feel like a part-time or even full-time job.

Unfortunately, stress can further compromise our digestion. Normally, if we are relaxed when we eat, the parasympathetic nervous system is activated, which allows us to "rest and digest." But if we are on high alert during eating because we are feeling ill or are worried about what we are eating, we tend to activate the sympathetic "fight or flight" system and do not digest food well. Stress also negatively affects the MMC, which may already be compromised in those with SIBO.

In addition to stress, there can be neurological symptoms such as brain fog, anxiety, poor memory, and depression. Gut bacteria produce hundreds of neurochemicals that support the brain in regulating mental health processes, and a bacterial imbalance can compromise these processes, which in turn affects moods, learning, and memory. For instance, up to 95 percent of our serotonin—the neurotransmitter largely responsible for regulating mood—is manufactured in the gut. If gut dysbiosis reduces how much serotonin is made or delivered to the brain through the vagus nerve, we may experience depression or anxiety.

A deficiency in vitamin B_{12} may also cause depression or mood issues. Histamine intolerance can also result in symptoms of brain fog, and changing one's diet may bring relief.

It is important to not just live with your mood changes but also check with a qualified health-care provider to run specific lab work and find out where deficiencies may exist, as well as find a SIBO diet that is helpful to you. It may be a multilayered journey to find out how SIBO is connected to specific neurological symptoms, but know that you are not alone in feeling the way you do.

YOU CAN FEEL BETTER

After reading about the many different forms of SIBO, you should have a greater understanding of your own symptoms and how they might be connected to SIBO. Although you have probably made great strides in living with your SIBO symptoms, this does not have to be your new normal, and you should not have to get used to being uncomfortable or in pain on a regular basis. This chapter discussed both possible short-term ways to mitigate symptoms and covered longer-term treatments.

The most important takeaway is that there are ways to feel better both now and in the long run. There is hope. Having hope is about not just having faith in getting better but also educating yourself so you know what you are up against and how to understand your options. In reading this book, you are supporting yourself in discerning your path, knowing how you got to where you are, and what your next steps forward look like.

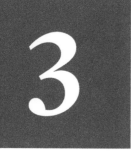

Diagnosing SIBO

MOST OF THE PEOPLE I SPEAK WITH ARE GRATEFUL TO finally get a SIBO diagnosis. They have frequently not been taken seriously by doctors, told they cannot be helped, or been misdiagnosed. Many have undergone multiple invasive and sometimes expensive tests but have never been asked to take a SIBO test.

But what about after the diagnosis? Or if you do not have a diagnosis but suspect you have SIBO? Wherever you are now is okay. Receiving a diagnosis can be daunting, but there is hope for managing SIBO. In this chapter, I will walk you through what receiving a SIBO diagnosis looks like and outline your next steps for moving forward.

How to Diagnose SIBO

The symptoms of SIBO are frequently gastrointestinal in nature, and such issues are often considered socially shameful (even though they certainly are not). So it is not surprising that many people do not want to speak to a doctor about them. When my own SIBO symptoms began to worsen, it was confusing. When I ate healthy items like salads for lunch, I would feel awful, with bowel cramping and small, frequent, irritated bowel movements. I did not understand why I started having diarrhea and why so many foods did not agree with me. I considered myself healthy and did not know what I was doing wrong to cause such unpleasant symptoms. I kept hoping it would get better, but when I became more ill over time, I finally decided to see a doctor. I think my scenario is fairly typical. We often blame ourselves for our symptoms and do not seek the help we need until we have exhausted all other options.

When people do seek treatment, they still may not receive the help they need. Not all doctors know about SIBO or believe it is a legitimate issue because it is still relatively new in the mainstream medical community. With SIBO, it is paramount to understand the underlying cause, and that identifying an underlying cause does not mean that SIBO itself does not exist on top of it. The doctors who do recognize SIBO are not always clear on treatment. They may prescribe an antibiotic that is not SIBO-specific, or they may assume that a round of antibiotics will clear a patient's overgrowth without first conducting and interpreting a test to see if their patient has a large or small overgrowth. The road to diagnosis can be frustrating for some, but scientific research on SIBO continues to be conducted and more information is becoming available daily. Awareness continues to grow, so there is hope for those newly diagnosed or still suffering.

Tests for SIBO can be helpful to establish an official medical diagnosis, but before you request testing or follow your doctor's recommendation to conduct them, it is important to review your symptoms.

Although you can be diagnosed only by a doctor, these symptoms may indicate you have SIBO:

- You have diarrhea, constipation, gas, or bloating.

- Your symptoms started or worsened after food poisoning, stomach flu, surgery, or heavy antibiotic, opiate, or proton-pump inhibitor (PPI) use.

- You experience constipation and need to use high doses of magnesium, vitamin C, laxatives, or enemas to have regular bowel movements.

- You have undesired weight loss or weight gain, nutritional deficiencies (including chronic B_{12} deficiency), low ferritin, or anemia that cannot be attributed to other causes.

- You react poorly to high-fiber or high-FODMAP foods.

- You react to foods that you used to be able to consume without any issues.

- Changing your diet by removing dairy or gluten has not made a discernible difference in your symptoms.

- You have adopted a very restrictive diet to reduce your symptoms.

- Taking antibiotics for other ailments gave you respite from your symptoms.

- You have experienced mental health changes such as increased anxiety.

Not everyone's symptoms fit into this picture, but it is important for you to discuss your symptoms with your doctor in addition to taking a SIBO test.

Testing is an important part of an official SIBO diagnosis. Let's discuss the tests for SIBO and SIBO-related issues and the efficacy of each.

BREATH TEST

A hydrogen-and-methane breath test is generally considered the standard test to diagnose SIBO. Breath tests are available with either glucose or lactulose as the substrate. After a prep period with a specific prep diet and an overnight fast, the first breath sample is collected. Then the substrate is taken with water, and nine more breath samples are collected, for a total of 10 tubes. The air in the tubes is measured for hydrogen and methane gases. QuinTron is the largest manufacturer of the breath test, and in my practice, I recommend labs that offer its lactulose breath test.

SMALL-BOWEL ASPIRATE TEST

A small-bowel aspirate test, specifically a duodenal aspirate culture, can be collected during an upper endoscopy. However, since an endoscopy is a somewhat invasive procedure and requires anesthesia, this test is not commonly recommended. There is also a possibility of a false negative if the sample is not large enough or if the area from which the culture is taken does not contain an overgrowth, even if other parts of the jejunum or duodenum do contain one.

STOOL TEST

Stool tests use a feces sample to diagnose issues or infections in the large intestine, such as bacterial dysbiosis (an imbalance of large-intestine bacteria), a large-intestine bacterial overgrowth (LIBO), parasites, or large-intestine fungal overgrowth (LIFO). However, stool tests cannot determine if an overgrowth exists in the small intestine.

URINE ORGANIC ACID TEST

There are no scientific studies showing that organic acid tests should be used to diagnose SIBO. This test measures key metabolites in the urine, but they cannot be connected to specific bacteria or fungal markers.

THE INS AND OUTS OF BREATH TESTING

Even though a breath test is the best one currently for diagnosing SIBO, some people might not be able to complete one. It can be challenging for younger children, since there is a specific way to collect the breath that takes attention to detail. For some, the substrate (glucose or lactulose) may cause gastric upset. In most people, the symptoms are minimal, but for some, they can be enough that they may not want to take the test again. Since those with diabetes or other health conditions may not be able to complete a 12-hour fast before the test, taking the breath test may not be an option for them. For people with extreme constipation, taking the test can also be challenging since all laxatives must be stopped for four days before the test.

As long as the preparatory diet and general guidelines are followed, the breath test should be valid. When discussing the breath test results with your doctor, it is important to remember that some doctors examine the gas results of the first 90 minutes, whereas some look at the first 120 minutes. The 120-minute mark is typically thought to be the transition between the small and large intestine.

Most labs have slightly different ways of presenting test results, and in the end, it is up to the doctor to interpret the results and make a diagnosis. A 2017 breath test consensus brought together multiple SIBO-focused doctors, and they deemed a rise greater or equal to 20 ppm (parts per million) of hydrogen during a lactulose or glucose breath test to be a positive diagnosis for SIBO. Methane levels above or equal to 10 ppm are also considered positive.

If a SIBO diagnosis is given and a treatment is undertaken, it is useful to test again after the treatment is complete. With larger overgrowths, one round of treatment may not completely remove them. So it is helpful to see how much the numbers went down and how the person reacted to specific treatments. This, along with any symptoms that occurred during treatment, can guide both the doctor and the patient in deciding if it is helpful to do a second round of the same treatment or switch to a different one. Thus, some people will take a SIBO test after each treatment and others may do one less frequently.

For those with chronic SIBO, testing and focusing only on the test numbers rather than going by the actual symptoms can trigger anxiety and distress. It may be helpful emotionally to take a break from testing. In my experience, since my overgrowth was large, I took multiple SIBO tests to see how I was reacting to different rounds of antibiotics. After about two years and many rounds of treatments, I received a negative SIBO test. But a year later, another test came back with positive results. At that point, I took a break from testing because I felt too much at the mercy of numbers.

I paid attention to my diet, continued to make adjustments, and worked with doctors on some associated issues, including parasites and yeast overgrowth. I have not taken a full SIBO test in the last few years, but I did recently take a spot test for methane (which is just one breath, without consuming a substrate), and I was negative for methane. I also continue to largely exclude gluten, dairy, and some grains from my diet, which is helpful to me, but it is not necessarily for everyone. Otherwise, I try to make my diet as diverse as possible to support my microbiome, and I no longer react negatively to high-FODMAP foods.

At this point, my lack of symptoms is enough evidence for me to believe that I no longer have SIBO. I do not think I would be where I am now if I had not gone through multiple rounds of treatment, but it was also important for me to address it in a different way once the size of the overgrowth had receded.

What Does a SIBO Diagnosis Mean?

Getting a positive diagnosis for SIBO can be both a relief and heart-wrenching. But the good news is that SIBO is manageable, and many people start feeling better after beginning treatment and incorporating dietary changes. A more restrictive diet is really meant to be a shorter-term modification; even when you are on a diet, you should still find ways to enjoy food with family and friends. It is important to continue to enjoy your food and your life while dealing with SIBO and its related treatments. You may feel embarrassed or ashamed of your symptoms, but you do not need to be. Just as with any health issue, having a support network is key to not feeling alone as well as getting validation.

Although statistics on recovery from SIBO are not available at this time, it is generally thought that about one-third of SIBO cases are more easily resolved and the other two-thirds have a longer journey. This might be because of underlying causes or multiple gastrointestinal issues at the same time.

When I was diagnosed many years ago, I had never heard of SIBO, but the thought of completely changing my diet made me angry and sad. I have always been someone who loves food and sharing community around a table, so it felt like I was being asked to change who I was. Part of my learning was to discover how to connect with people away from food or while eating the food that supported me.

Because I started on the specific carbohydrate diet (SCD), which requires fanatical adherence, I did not do a lot of testing outside of that one diet. In retrospect, I wish I had not bought into the fear around food and would have tested more things outside of that very restricted diet. At a later point, I did just that, and then I began to really understand more about my body's cues when specific foods did or did not agree with me. You will, too. The recipes in this book are designed to support your digestive system while still allowing you to enjoy your food.

What to Expect from Your GI Doctor

When you visit a doctor who works with SIBO patients, most doctors will review the lab work and discuss your symptoms and medical history. Some will do a physical exam, which can be helpful in discovering a hiatal hernia or an ileocecal valve dysfunction, either of which may be connected to SIBO. If the doctor suspects you have SIBO, a test will likely be ordered for you. Once the results are available, your doctor should talk about the size of your overgrowth and if a particular SIBO treatment is recommended in relation to your test results. If you already have a test result and have seen other doctors in the past, this doctor will likely want more information about your particular treatments, your reactions to them, if you tested again afterward, and how your symptoms changed over time. Either way, many doctors will recommend a SIBO-friendly diet to see if it helps mitigate some of your symptoms.

If you are visiting a doctor who is not familiar with SIBO or has seen only a handful of patients with SIBO, it is helpful to bring in your own research and a list of possible treatment options. I recommend viewing Dr. Allison Siebecker's website, SiboInfo.com, as it lists many different treatments in specific dosages and lengths of time. Each doctor may have a slightly different approach, but it is helpful to have some understanding of these general practices when you go in.

There is certainly a happy medium where research is concerned. You want to know and understand enough to discuss SIBO with your doctor and even direct them if they are new to treating the condition. However, because many patients tend to be in a heightened state of anxiety and hypervigilance, they look up every single comment or suggestion for treating SIBO from both doctors and patients on the Internet and want to try everything—often all at once. Most health-care providers advise against that, as it is important to know what is working, and a "kitchen sink" approach could result in not only increased symptoms but a step backward. Remember, research is powerful, but focusing on actual studies and data is crucial. Look for repetition in the information you read, learn which researchers or health-care providers are trustworthy, and know when to take a step back and take a break from research.

In general, if you are seeing a doctor who does not believe in SIBO, I recommend you find one who does. It is hard enough to be sick without also feeling like your doctor is not curious about and invested in your health. It will also put you in a better place to receive SIBO-specific treatment and to know that your doctor has worked with SIBO patients before, which can relieve some anxiety.

If you do not feel like you are making headway with your doctor, it is important to assess why. It is not a matter of blaming yourself or the doctor, but it is vital to note what is not being addressed. Have you discussed your underlying cause? Is your diet mitigating some of your symptoms? Working through SIBO, especially if there are multiple concurrent issues, can take time and patience. Trust your instincts on whether your doctor has your best interests in mind and remember that they may not have all the answers. It is often helpful, when possible, to have a team of people to address SIBO. This might include a doctor, a nutritionist, a mental health counselor, a bodywork therapist, and others. You might see some of these people regularly, whereas others may require less frequent visits. It is really a matter of discovering what works best for you. It is your health, and ultimately you are in charge of it.

What It Means to Self-Diagnose SIBO

If you have self-diagnosed by checking your symptoms and researching online, it is important to be able to tell your doctor why you feel you have SIBO. Make sure you are clear and concise in your reasoning, and it very well may help you save time on the way to a diagnosis.

A SIBO diagnosis should typically be performed by a doctor, but if you do not have access to health care, lack SIBO-literate doctors in your area, or think you have been misdiagnosed, you may feel that the only choice you have is to self-diagnose.

Before you do so, I recommend trying to find a SIBO-literate doctor or other health-care provider who provides long-distance consultations. They will not be able to diagnose you, but they can discuss your case with you. It is often helpful to have an outside viewpoint from an educated professional. There are lists of SIBO-literate health-care providers throughout the United States (see the Resources section on page 164 for more information).

If you absolutely cannot find a doctor, then I recommend you work with a health professional who can be a part of your support system along your journey. Nutritionists and health coaches are not able to diagnose or treat, but they can collaborate with you in other important and helpful ways.

The Condition versus the Cause

Typically, SIBO is not a condition that is seen in isolation but rather the result of an underlying cause. Sometimes it takes some work to identify that cause, and some people will never know with certainty. Even if you do not know your underlying cause, it is still important to deal with the SIBO itself, so getting a diagnosis is definitely a step in the right direction.

It can be especially difficult to determine an underlying cause if patients have had gastrointestinal symptoms their whole life or if they have multiple risk factors. However, we know that in many cases, the MMC has been compromised to a certain extent and that supporting it through prokinetics after a treatment is an important part of preventing SIBO recurrence. So is diet, as it may relieve symptoms and accompanying inflammation, and adjusting it can help set the stage for healing.

Speak Up about SIBO

For most people, SIBO affects what and how they eat. Dealing with its symptoms affects daily life, so it is important to speak up about SIBO and let people know how your daily routines and needs have changed. Verbalizing your experience also helps others know they can talk about their own experiences, and that helps demystify digestive issues. It can also help you grow your network of supportive people around you.

If you are comfortable with and want to talk about the specific symptoms you are having, it is helpful to have several people with whom you can be totally candid. It might also be useful to let them know the basics about SIBO and what your journey may look like, if you have any indication.

As for those with whom you are not as close, it may be helpful to explain to them how your life has changed even if you do not want to discuss individual symptoms. For example, you may want to tell your employer that you will be bringing your own lunch for potlucks or catered events, or that you will be taking more sick time for medical appointments.

And for those whom you do not know at all, it is still important to understand your boundaries at any given time and be ready to address inappropriate questions or observations. Because health and nutrition are such major parts of our culture, many people love to talk about different diets, especially if they think it pertains to weight loss. I was at a birthday function once and was eating only one item. Someone I did not know suggested I was on a weight-loss diet and I told her I was not, even though what I was eating was not her business. She brought it up a second time, so I calmly told her I had SIBO and this was the only item I could eat without there being gastrointestinal repercussions. We talked a little bit about my situation, and she clearly felt bad for bringing it up. Hopefully, I was able to educate her a little bit, and perhaps in the future, she will be more sensitive.

I have many stories where people may have had good intentions but were not always kind or polite in their reactions to or commentary on what I was eating. I always appreciated when someone was clearly worried about my health and truly showed compassion. It was more challenging when I received congratulatory comments about my weight loss from people who did not know or care that I had lost weight because I was sick.

Through my own health journey, I learned to set my boundaries. It is important to know that regardless of whom you are speaking to, there is nothing to be ashamed of in regard to having SIBO, and you get to decide what is appropriate to talk about and share.

Find Your SIBO Support Group

When you have SIBO, it is important to find support within your current community and also to create a new one with those who share similar struggles.

Your partner, family, or friends may not have SIBO, but they can still show concern for you and will most likely want to learn about what you are going through. You can talk to them about the parameters of your therapeutic diet, how your medical appointments are going, or what your course of treatment will be. Of course, no one wants to talk about SIBO all the time, and it is important for both you and your community to take a break from it. But sharing your fears, symptoms, efforts, and progress are important parts of the healing process, as is not feeling alone.

Creating a community with those who have or have had SIBO can also be helpful emotionally and educationally. There are Facebook and other online groups as well as in-person support groups for SIBO. For online groups, I suggest finding a moderated group that does not allow others to sell their services and posts only supportive comments. No one should be diagnosing or suggesting treatment online, but it can be very helpful to hear someone else's story and what worked for them. You can also share your own journey and be a comfort and resource to others. Please see the Resources section on page 164 for more information on online groups.

You Aren't Alone

Even if you have not realized it yet, you are already part of a community of people who have been diagnosed with or are learning more about SIBO. Although it may not be a club you wanted to become a member of, it is important that you are educating yourself about SIBO, including the steps to testing and diagnosis. It is also important to know that you are not alone. By joining SIBO support groups and allowing your community to support you, you will meet people who lift you up, act as your lighthouse, and give you information that makes a world of difference in your health. Even though you may feel isolated right now, you are taking the first steps in making connections, with both yourself and others out there who are also beginning their own healing journeys.

4

Treating SIBO

ALTHOUGH OFFICIAL SIBO STATISTICS ON RECURRENCE are not available, we know that within the SIBO community, many patients have experienced one after getting a negative test result. That may be because more doctors are learning what SIBO is and how to treat it. And since some doctors do not recommend retesting after treatment, it is possible that in some cases the overgrowth was never actually eradicated.

Once the SIBO is gone, it is also important to address the underlying cause, support a gut healing phase with prokinetics, and initiate food reintroduction after a more restricted diet. Some people may have ongoing SIBO because of underlying causes or anatomical differences. But this should be a much smaller subset of people.

This chapter will review the different treatments for SIBO as well as steps to mitigate symptoms, including diet and lifestyle changes. It is of the utmost importance that you be informed of your options so you can partner with your doctor to determine the right course of treatment specific to you.

Know Your Options, Have Patience, and Remain Positive

Typically, a SIBO treatment involves multiple components. They may include diet and lifestyle changes, herbal or pharmaceutical medications, an elemental diet, and bodywork. It is important to put together a health-care team who can address all of your medical needs. Remember, YOU are the most important member of your team. You may be the patient, but you also know yourself better than anyone else, and it is important to support yourself in every way possible, as well as being your own best advocate.

Dietary Changes: Food is so connected to not only our social lives but also our physical and emotional states. An SIBO-friendly diet is typically lower in fermentable carbohydrates because bacterial overgrowths feed on such foods, which increases symptoms. For people with very minor overgrowths, dietary changes may be enough to eliminate their SIBO. For most people, dietary changes alone will not eradicate SIBO, but they can greatly reduce symptoms and set the stage for healing.

Lifestyle Changes: Most people need to make some at least temporary lifestyle changes while they have SIBO, if not permanent changes. Many people experience increased anxiety and stress from having to modify their diet and spend more time at medical appointments, cooking, and researching. Although this is understandable, your body will heal better if it gets enough rest and has continual chances to be in a parasympathetic (rest-and-digest) state. It has been my experience with both myself and my clients that many of us with SIBO tend to be go-getters who have a propensity to take on too much. If that sounds like you, it might be time to reevaluate your schedule and your sources of stress to see what you can change.

Elemental Diet: The elemental diet is not a diet to relieve symptoms; it is specifically considered a treatment. The elemental diet involves a premixed or homemade formula that is the only thing you consume for two to three weeks. Dr. Allison Siebecker has created a homemade formula that is available on her website (see the Resources section on page 164), and premade options are available, too. The formula gives you everything your body needs to survive, including carbohydrates, protein in the form of amino acids, fat, and necessary nutrients. But because it is elemental and no other food is consumed, it does not feed an over-growth. Instead of killing bacteria like an antibiotic, the elemental diet starves bacteria to remove the overgrowth.

Medication: Pharmaceutical antibiotics can be prescribed only by med-ical professionals and should be taken only under the care of a licensed provider. Typically, rifaximin (Xifaxan is the generic name) is given for all cases of SIBO, and neomycin or metronidazole (Flagyl) is added for cases where constipation is present. Typical dosing for these antibiot-ics is listed on Dr. Siebecker's website (see the Resources section on page 164). A typical course of rifaximin is 10 to 14 days.

Rifaximin may be the preferred pharmaceutical antibiotic for many doctors because it is local to the intestine and not a systemic antibiotic, so patients do not seem to become resistant to it. If patients respond well to it once, they tend to do so again. However, if its cost is not cov-ered by insurance, it can be very expensive.

Natural Remedies: Even though herbal antibiotics and antimicrobials can be obtained without a prescription, you should still discuss your specific treatment with your doctor and take herbal remedies only under their advisement. In specific doses, they do the same thing as a pharmaceutical antibiotic: kill bacteria. They are preferred by some licensed naturo-pathic doctors, although their efficacy also depends on what the patient responds to. A 2014 study by Johns Hopkins University found that herbal antibiotics were just as successful as rifaximin in treating SIBO.

Herbals can be taken as a multiherbal combination contained in one capsule or as individual herbs. Those who are more sensitive can start with one herb in a smaller dose, then ramp up to the regular dose over time before adding the next herb, and so on. In this scenario, if one herb is not tolerated, it can be identified and removed rather than stopping an entire treatment protocol.

The Elemental Diet

Some people love the elemental diet because they do not have to worry about what they are eating, and they often feel less symptomatic and may have more energy because the formula is easy to absorb.

Others have found the diet to be challenging because they are consuming only a beverage for all of their meals, are not able to socialize around meals for two to three weeks, or get tired of the taste. Many people lose weight while they are on the elemental diet, so it is not necessarily recommended for those who are already underweight.

Most people experience food cravings, but their desire to feel better typically overrides their longing for a specific food. Die-off, or a Jarisch-Herxheimer reaction, is also fairly common. The bacteria release endotoxins as they die off, causing flu-like symptoms that may include fatigue, joint pain, headaches, nausea, diarrhea, or constipation. These symptoms tend to subside after a couple of days for most people. If possible, it is helpful to have a flexible schedule when you start the diet in case a day off from work, school, or other obligations is necessary, but most people experience lighter symptoms.

A 2004 study found that the elemental diet was highly successful in eradicating SIBO. Out of 93 patients, 80 percent had a normal breath test after two weeks on the elemental diet. Those who did not continued for a third week. Of that subset, 85 percent experienced a normal breath test after the third week. The elemental diet often brings down a higher overgrowth more effectively than a round of herbal or pharmaceutical antibiotics. So for those with higher breath-test numbers, starting with the elemental diet may be an efficient course of action.

After the elemental diet, solid food should be reintroduced slowly. The digestion process needs to be restarted, so it is helpful to ease into it with broths, purées, soups, and stews for a couple of days and then add in more solid foods over time.

Talk to your health-care provider about whether the elemental diet is the right option for you.

Bodywork: Adhesions (scar tissue) from surgeries or radiation therapy may be an underlying cause of SIBO. Visceral manipulation, specialized physical therapy, or abdominal massage can be an important part of SIBO treatment for some people.

Your Health-Care Team: Your health-care team may include a doctor, nutritionist, bodyworker, mental health counselor, and health coach. No matter who you put on your team, it is important to utilize them to the fullest extent. Remember, these are people who are used to talking about bowel movements and a variety of symptoms, so do not be shy in sharing your questions, challenges, and frustrations.

Managing SIBO through Diet

With SIBO, there is no "one size fits all," and that goes for both antibiotics and dietary changes. Everyone will have different reactions to food. Some people do very poorly with rice, potatoes, and other higher-starch items, whereas others are fine with them and find that they prevent unwanted weight loss. Some people cannot eat any raw fruits and vegetables without undigested food appearing in their stools or bowel cramping, but others are fine with raw produce. That is why it is so important to tailor the diet to suit your preferences and tolerances and get professional support if and when you need it.

Here are some recommendations for anyone starting a SIBO diet:

- For most people, a SIBO diet will help mitigate symptoms. It is not typically used as a primary treatment for SIBO.

- If you are not sure which foods you tolerate, start with ones that are easy to digest, such as peeled, seeded, and well-cooked fruits and vegetables. Try vegetables mashed, puréed, or in soups. That is not to say you can never enjoy a salad again, but try smaller side salads and note any accompanying symptoms.

- Allow four to five hours in between meals to support the MMC. Some people may need to eat more often because of malabsorption or blood sugar issues; if this is your case, try to eat a snack closer to a mealtime. For instance, if you eat breakfast at 8 a.m., wait until at least 11 a.m. for a snack, and then have your lunch at 12 p.m. so that you leave at least three hours between eating. Over time, you may be able to further space out your eating, but remember that your immediate health should come first. You should not experience dizziness, headaches, or any other drastic symptoms from not eating for three hours. Try to distinguish between a normal "Oh, I am getting hungry" response versus one that is more critical.

- If you are moving away from a higher-carb, processed-food diet, it is likely that you will experience some carbohydrate cravings. This is normal and they will decrease over time. But do not overly restrict yourself; find lower-carb treats that you think are delicious.

- Take snacks or meals with you if you will be gone for all or part of a day. Timelines shift and you never know when you will be hungry or if you will not be able to get home for a meal.

- Eat the highest-quality food you can afford. Review the produce shopping guides put out by the Environmental Working Group (see the Resources section on page 164) to see which fruits and vegetables are more likely to contain high pesticide residues. Buy organic for the foods on the Dirty Dozen™ list and review the Clean Fifteen™ list for the produce that is safe to buy in conventional form. Whenever possible, buy grass-fed, free-range meat and eggs. Since meat is at the top of the food chain, the level of toxins you can get from conventionally raised animals that have eaten genetically modified organisms (GMOs) or conventionally grown feed is significant. Buy more affordable cuts of meat (such as roasts) to save money. You can also buy them in bulk and freeze them as needed.

- If you experience rapid or unwanted weight loss, try eating combinations of fat and carbohydrates to retain weight. If you tolerate white rice, white potato, white bread, or other grains and higher-starch vegetables, make sure to eat a serving with each meal.

- Part of discovering what you can tolerate is trying new foods and then seeing if they agree with you. This can be a challenging process, but it should ultimately give you a more diverse diet that supports your microbiome as well as your overall health. Be aware of both the amount and frequency in relation to what you are eating. Maybe you can handle a half cup of rice once a day without problems, but a full cup of rice twice a day causes symptoms. This is just one example, and the specifics will be different for everyone.

- If it does not bring up undue anxiety, it can be helpful to keep a diary of foods, symptoms, and bowel movements for a short time. Reviewing the food diary with your nutritionist or other health-care professional can help you ascertain which foods may be connected to ongoing symptoms.

- If you have a history of disordered eating or a diagnosed eating disorder, be sure your health-care providers know. Since SIBO diets can be restrictive, they may trigger disordered eating patterns. Work with a qualified nutritionist or mental health professional if these patterns come up for you.

- Many doctors recommend that their patients add in some higher-FODMAP foods during a SIBO treatment (except during the elemental diet). The thinking is that you feed the bacteria so they do not "hibernate" but instead are active and therefore ready to be eliminated by the antibiotic. This is not an invitation to get pizza, beer, and ice cream—rather, it is a time to add a couple of higher-FODMAP foods that you have been missing but are unlikely to put you into a flare state.

- In addition to SIBO, some people experience histamine, sulfur, oxalate, or salicylate sensitivity. Further dietary modifications may be needed to relieve related symptoms.

- Review additional information and links in the Resources section on page 164.

MANAGING SIBO THROUGH DIET: THE LOW-FODMAP DIET

- FODMAP stands for fermentable oligosaccharides, disaccharides, monosaccharides, and polyols. FODMAPs are typically a healthy part of one's diet, but when you have SIBO, these fermentable foods can feed a bacterial overgrowth, which in turn causes symptoms.

- Because the low-FODMAP diet excludes fermentable foods but does not exclude polysaccharides like starchier foods, the low-FODMAP diet suits those with mild to moderate symptoms.

- This diet includes grains and starchier items, so it can be very helpful to those experiencing unwanted weight loss.

- The low-FODMAP diet has been studied and proven to be beneficial for those with IBS. Since up to 84 percent of people with IBS also have SIBO, it is reasonable to expect that the diet will help many people with SIBO. Not everyone with SIBO reacts to high-FODMAP foods, but many do.

- Numerous FODMAP lists exist on the Internet, but many are out of date or incorrect. I recommend using the Monash University FODMAP diet app. Monash University continually conducts scientific testing to ascertain FODMAP levels in particular foods. The app is updated on an ongoing basis, is easy to use, and is inexpensive (see the Resources section on page 164).

- The low-FODMAP diet does not include a phased approach, but books like my first one, *The SIBO Diet Plan*, offer meal plans that add new foods over time.

- Since high-FODMAP foods are typically a healthy part of the diet, it is not recommended to stay on a low-FODMAP diet on an ongoing basis.

MANAGING SIBO THROUGH DIET: SCD

- The specific carbohydrate diet (SCD) eliminates polysaccharides from the diet but does not exclude FODMAPs. Therefore, the SCD is best for someone who does not react to FODMAPs but may be reacting to other carbohydrates.

- The SCD has been studied for people with irritable bowel disease, which includes ulcerative colitis and Crohn's disease. However, its efficacy has not been studied for SIBO.

- The diet has a list of "legal" and "illegal" foods, which suggests fanatical adherence. These terms and mind-set could be triggering for someone with an eating disorder or someone who is prone to disordered eating.

MANAGING SIBO THROUGH DIET: THE SIBO SPECIFIC FOOD GUIDE

- The SIBO Specific Food Guide (SSFG) was created by Dr. Allison Siebecker and is a combination of the low-FODMAP, SCD, and Dr. Siebecker's clinical experience. Since the SSFG is more restrictive, people with more severe symptoms will benefit the most from it.

- This diet can and should be customized, especially for anyone who will be on it for a longer time. Trying foods outside of the "green/less fermentable" column is recommended.

MANAGING SIBO THROUGH DIET: THE BI-PHASIC DIET

- The SIBO Bi-Phasic Diet (BPD), created by Dr. Nirala Jacobi, is based on Dr. Siebecker's SSFG, but it has some food modifications and uses a two-phase approach to limit bacterial die-off reactions.

- Because this diet combines both SCD and low-FODMAP elements and is additionally more restrictive in its first phase, it is well-suited to those with severe symptoms.

- This diet incorporates some grains like rice or quinoa in the first phase, semirestricted, and later portions of the diet, so it may be helpful for those who benefit from a more restrictive diet but still need some starchy foods to maintain their weight or energy level.

MANAGING SIBO THROUGH DIET: THE CEDARS-SINAI DIET (CSD)

- The goal of the Cedars-Sinai Medical Center's Low Fermentation Diet is for people who want to still feel like they can eat out and have a social life. Therefore, it is helpful for people who prefer more freedom and have milder symptoms.

- The diet recommends consuming lactose-free dairy (excluding yogurt); simple carbohydrates like rice, potatoes, sweet potatoes, and white bread; meat; fruit; eggs; mushrooms; anything that grows underground, such as onions, garlic, beets, carrots, and turnips; and fruit-type vegetables such as peppers, tomatoes, cucumbers, zucchini, squash, and eggplant.

- The diet excludes lactose-containing dairy products, beans and legumes, cabbage, Brussels sprouts, broccoli, cauliflower, leafy greens, and indigestible sugars like xylitol, sorbitol, or sucralose.

- This diet is not a good choice for those who do not tolerate polysaccharides or high-FODMAP foods, as they will likely be more symptomatic while following this diet.

Moving On from a SIBO Diet

If you are making progress with bringing down your overgrowth, it can be helpful to stay on your diet to continue to alleviate symptoms. Once you receive a negative test result, continue your diet for another month and then begin to diversify it. If you are on a low-FODMAP diet, test foods that have only one specific FODMAP by themselves so you know which FODMAPs you tolerate and which ones you do not. For instance, both avocado and fresh yellow peaches, in certain amounts, contain higher levels of sorbitol. Testing several foods that have moderate or high amounts of sorbitol can help ascertain if you tolerate that specific FODMAP. In addition to the FODMAP, you need to examine the fiber level in certain foods if you are still not tolerating higher amounts of fiber.

If you have worked with your doctor and discovered that, because of your underlying cause or concurrent factors, you are far more likely to relapse or have SIBO on an ongoing basis, then you will want to adopt a modified diet long-term. This means you should continue to test and add foods to make your diet as diverse as possible, but you may need to leave out some moderate or high-FODMAP foods or other foods you may remain sensitive to, such as gluten or dairy.

Soothing Foods for SIBO

Regardless of the diet you choose to follow, here are the top five types of foods to avoid, the top six types to eat that often soothe SIBO symptoms, and the top nine foods you will need to assess on a case-by-case basis.

FOODS TO AVOID

Dirty Dozen™ Fruits and Vegetables: These are conventionally farmed fruits and vegetables that are included in the Dirty Dozen™ list from the Environmental Working Group (see page 161) and are known to have higher pesticide residues. These are unhealthy for everyone, but they can be especially detrimental for someone who is trying to recover from SIBO and is already in an inflamed state. Make sure to eat organic versions of these foods.

Processed or Low-Quality Foods: It is important to embrace a whole-food diet for overall health and for healing from SIBO. Processed foods often contain high levels of sugar, salt, gums, and food coloring. These ingredients do not support your health and may even cause symptoms.

Have Sympathy for Slipups

The SIBO road to recovery is often winding, and discovering what works for you foodwise can be challenging and frustrating. There may be times you have slipups or you try a new food and have a really negative reaction. This is common, and although it may cause you gastrointestinal distress, it can also be instructional. You will learn where and how you can safely eat out. If you are often going off your diet, or if it feels like it often makes you anxious or stressed, it may be time to make some changes. Maybe you need to go on a less restrictive diet, or you need to hire someone to help with cooking. It is important that the diet works for you and that you do not work for it. In the case of trying new foods, it is imperative to continue to diversify your diet. Testing new foods is like detective work. Your body is supporting you by giving you clues as to how it tolerates the new food. If you tend to be more sensitive, test foods in smaller amounts first. If you have a reaction, always get back to a neutral point before you try a new food. The most significant piece is to be kind to yourself. We all make mistakes, but what we take from them is what matters.

Snacks: When possible, leave four to five hours between meals so the MMC can perform its sweeping and cleansing wave through the small intestine. For many people with SIBO, their MMC is already impaired, so it is important to support it by fasting between meals.

Unhealthy Fats: Avoid canola oil, corn oil, sunflower oil, and partially hydrogenated vegetable oils. They tend to be heavily processed, are often genetically modified, and can contain pesticides.

Difficult-to-Digest Foods: When you start a SIBO diet, it is important to peel, seed, and cook all fruits and vegetables to make them easier to digest. Avoiding high-fiber foods is a must for most people, as they typically cause symptoms for those with SIBO.

FOODS TO EAT

Low-FODMAP Fruits and Vegetables: Eat peeled, seeded, well-cooked fruits and vegetables in items like compotes, soups, purées, and stews. If you are digesting your food well and do not see undigested pieces in your stool, try a side salad but keep raw foods to smaller amounts. Also, make sure they are softer, such as butter lettuce rather than kale.

Low-FODMAP Bone Broth: Bone broth is easily digestible and is rich in iron, vitamins A and K, selenium, zinc, manganese, and fatty acids. It can be used as a base for soups, gravies, and stews. It can also be used as cooking liquid for rice or consumed by itself.

Healthy Fats: Healthy fats are a necessary part of our diet and help us stay satiated between meals. They support blood sugar regulation, are anti-inflammatory, and support absorption of the fat-soluble vitamins A, D, E, and K. Try fats like organic ghee or butter from grass-fed cows, coconut oil, olive oil, avocado oil, or organic beef tallow. We also use sesame oil in some of the recipes as a finishing (uncooked) oil.

Fish and Seafood: Wild salmon, cod, sardines, scallops, shrimp, and tuna are among the healthiest seafoods available to us. They all contain anti-inflammatory omega-3 fatty acids.

Healthy Animal Protein: Studies have shown a significant difference between organic grass-fed beef and lamb and organic pasture-raised chicken and turkey versus those conventionally raised. For instance, grass-fed beef may contain over twice the amount of lutein and beta-carotene and more omega-3 fatty acids than conventionally raised beef. Consider buying from a local farm to get better-quality meat if that option is available. If not, look for organic and grass-fed meat in grocery stores. You can also buy meat in bulk and freeze it in portions.

Fresh Herbs and Spices: Herbs and spices, in smaller amounts, are often tolerated, and their addition easily changes the overall taste of a dish. Ginger, parsley, rosemary, sage, dill, basil, cinnamon, black pepper, and cumin are among the healthiest herbs and spices and are frequently used in recipes in this cookbook.

FOODS TO ASSESS

Caffeine: Caffeine can cause gastrointestinal distress. People love coffee, and I am no exception. But it is still important to see how caffeine and coffee in particular are affecting you. It may be helpful to take coffee out of your diet for a week or two and then reintroduce it. After switching over to decaf, I realized that caffeine was contributing to both my GI distress and my anxiety.

Alcohol: Alcohol may cause stomach upset or gastrointestinal symptoms in many people. I find that people with SIBO often do not tolerate it well. That does not mean you can't ever sip a glass of wine or enjoy a low-FODMAP alcoholic beverage, but make sure you assess how it affects you.

Eggs: The proteins in egg whites can be hard to digest, and people with fat malabsorption may not do well with egg yolks. It is helpful to test the whites and yolks separately to see how you react. Some people also find the eggs in baked goods are easier to digest than eggs cooked by themselves, like fried or scrambled eggs. I could not digest eggs well when I had SIBO, but now I am able to eat them again.

Dairy: High-FODMAP dairy contains lactose, which many people react to. Consider being cautious with low-FODMAP dairy, such as hard cheese and 24-hour yogurt. The milk proteins casein and whey may be hard for some people to digest. However, if you do not notice an issue, keep them in your diet, as they are a great source of healthy fat.

Fructose: Some people with SIBO (but not all) will have fructose malabsorption. If you do not, you can add moderate- and high-fructose items to your diet. Test foods such as sun-dried tomatoes, mango, and canned artichoke hearts to see if you react. Check the Monash University FODMAP app (see the Resources section on page 164) for fructose amounts.

Fat: Fat is a healthy, necessary part of our diet, but those with fat malabsorption (steatorrhea) may experience nausea after eating fat and see an oil slick in the toilet after a bowel movement. Enzymes, which are commonly used to help digest fat, include ox bile, lipase, and amylase. See your doctor to discuss your particular situation.

Nuts and Seeds: Nuts and seeds have numerous health benefits but can be hard to digest, particularly in larger amounts. If you are consuming larger quantities of mixed nuts or almond-flour baked goods, note how you feel after you eat them. I recommend consuming them in smaller portions.

Coconut: Some people tolerate coconut very well and find it to be a helpful addition to diversify their diet because they can use coconut oil, coconut milk, or coconut meat in many recipes. But at least half of my clients do not tolerate it at all, except maybe coconut oil. Make sure to note your symptoms when eating foods containing coconut and see how you feel.

Resistant Starch: Resistant starch is starch that does not break down and instead feeds our bacteria. This is typically good for us, but not in the case of an overgrowth. Once starchy foods like rice or potato are cooked and then cooled, the starch changes and becomes resistant starch. So some people will find rice easy to digest the first time it is cooked but may not tolerate it once it has cooled and been reheated. Most of my clients seem to tolerate resistant starch and do not notice symptoms, but some people certainly do.

A New Relationship with Food for a Healthy Gut

When you have SIBO, so much changes—your diet, the way you interact with food, and the way you socialize. It is important to take time to reflect on how to make these changes positive and continue to connect with food and those you care about in life-affirming ways.

Here are some things to consider as your relationship with food changes.

- Practice good food hygiene, including eating your food slowly, chewing your food well, and, when possible, dining with those whom you care about.

- For those who do not enjoy cooking or do not have time to cook, consider hiring a part-time personal chef or talk to a meal service to see if they can create meals to your specifications. It is often cheaper than you would think, and many people are looking to get more experience working with those on a therapeutic diet.

- If you are feeling like you are at war with food and your body, it is important to shift your perspective. Before each meal, take some time for yourself to silently (or out loud, if you prefer) thank the people who contributed to getting the food to you (that includes farmers, truck drivers, and grocery store clerks). Remind yourself that it is important to try new foods. If you experience symptoms, it is your body's way of helping you by giving you information. Take three deep breaths and feel your feet grounded on the floor before you begin eating. The more you can relax and mentally be in the present, the more you will enjoy eating and the better you will digest your food.

- If you have done a lot of Internet research, found lots of contradicting information, and now you feel like nothing is good for you or will work in your diet, you need to question your beliefs and your mind-set. It may be time to leave the research behind, go back to your food diary, and figure out what is good for *you* in particular.

- When I was on a very restrictive SIBO diet, I used to have dreams of eating things like doughnuts or cake, only to realize in my dream that I was not supposed to be eating them. I would wake up feeling guilty about something I had not even been able to enjoy. It is so important to make sure you do have food you enjoy. For example, many people do well with a little dark chocolate, and there are recipes for desserts in this book. Or if you have low-grade symptoms, you may be able to get away with having a bite or two of something not on your diet without ramifications. Make sure to try different foods and recipes that delight you.

- It is important to find new ways to connect with those you love. Instead of meeting out somewhere for a drink or dinner, try going for walks, crafting together, inviting someone over for a home-cooked meal, running errands together, or making a SIBO-friendly recipe together. It is lovely to connect for a meal, but it does not mean you always have to go out to a restaurant to eat.

- For parties, bring something you can eat yourself if possible. If you are not tolerating or do not want alcohol, try some sparkling water with lime.

- Before going out to eat, look at the menu in advance to see if there is something you know will be safe. If there is not, call the chef in the early afternoon before dinner service. Let them know when you will be in and that you would like a specific protein (like a chicken breast or a steak) with one or two sides that you tolerate (like white rice and carrots). Ask them to use only oils that you tolerate and to season the meal with just salt and pepper. When you get to the restaurant, let your server know that you spoke with the chef in advance and that they have okayed your order. Once you find a couple of restaurants where you feel safe eating, life will be a little easier. Even when it is food that you could make yourself at home, it is often just nice to be out, and it opens you up for more socializing.

- Holidays can be a challenging time with multiple social outings and family functions. If you can be an active part of the cooking process, it will make things easier in the long run. Make sure you have several things available that you can eat so you don't get to the table and feel like there is nothing for you.

- There may be times you feel too overwhelmed, tired, or sick to get together for a holiday or social gathering. It is important to know that it is okay to say no and take care of yourself. There is a difference between isolating yourself and taking care of your body. Make sure you find a happy medium.

- Vacations take a bit of extra planning. Booking a hotel room or a house rental with a small kitchen can be really beneficial so that you will not be forced to eat out at every meal. Find a local grocery store and stock up on items that work for you. Also, look up restaurants in advance to identify places that fit your dietary needs.

- If you end up eating at a place where you know you will be going off your diet, try to do your best to let go and enjoy yourself. The more you can relax and consider it an experiment, the more likely it is to go well.

Reset Your Gut but Enjoy Your Life

The changes you make will be significant, and they will take time and energy. Give yourself leeway when you feel frustrated or tired and want to give up. Remind yourself that the seeds you are sowing will make a vast difference in your long-term health and well-being. Find wellness practices that help you reset and stay grounded. These can include practicing gratitude, deep breathing, and meditation. Many options are available, so try a variety of things and see what resonates with you. It is important to know that you can feel whole even while you are healing.

Eating SIBO-Friendly
Can Still Be Tasty

Changing your diet does not have to mean giving up flavor. Here are some SIBO-friendly substitutions.

Eggs: You can use an egg replacer in baked goods, such as flaxseeds or chia seeds. If you tolerate egg yolks but not the whites, two egg yolks can replace one full egg.

Yogurt: Try homemade 24-hour lactose-free yogurt (see the 24-Hour Yogurt with Lemon-Berry Compote recipe on page 64). If you buy store-bought lactose-free yogurt, some will have gums, so check the label.

Onions: Onions are high-FODMAP and many people do not tolerate them. The green portions of scallions and chives can be used in dishes instead.

Garlic: Garlic is high-FOMDAP and many people are sensitive to it. To still get a garlicky flavor, you can sauté whole cloves in oil and then remove and discard them. Garlic-infused oil is also widely available. See the Resources section on page 164 for specific brands.

Soy Sauce: If you are avoiding gluten but tolerate soy, you can easily substitute tamari, which is gluten-free, for soy sauce. If you do not tolerate soy, you can easily substitute coconut aminos in a 1:1 ratio for soy sauce or tamari.

Pasta: Plain white rice noodles can be a substitute for spaghetti, and there are also some low-FODMAP pastas available. Spaghetti squash or spiralized "vegetable noodles" are also a great substitute.

Bread: If you tolerate gluten, white sourdough bread is recommended, but if not, white gluten-free bread can be tried to see if it is tolerated. There are also almond-flour bread recipes available online.

You Can Do This

We have reviewed a wealth of SIBO information in this chapter, including the ways to treat it, how dietary changes can help, what the diets look like, how to use them to your advantage, and tips for making them work for you. Take time with this process and come back and review this when things feel like they are not working. Remember, this whole process is a work in progress and you are doing the very best you can. When you need to, seek help from your medical team, including your doctor, nutritionist, or mental health counselor.

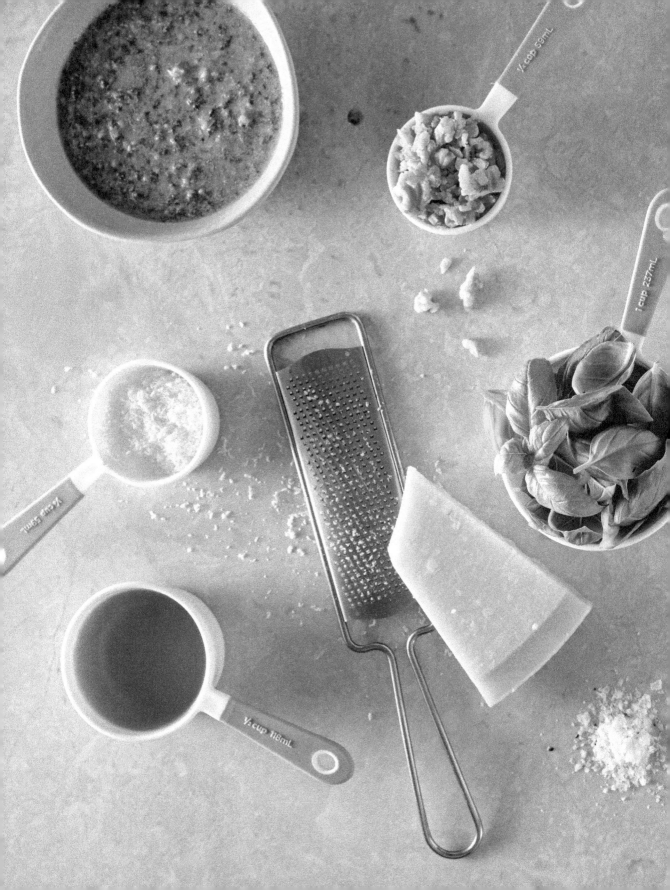

PART TWO
The Recipes

Eating is such an important part of our lives, and you should still be able to enjoy delicious food even if you have SIBO. These 50 recipes are designed to be healthy and easy to digest, with simple ingredients. They all fit into a FODMAP diet and are categorized as dairy-free, gluten-free, nut-free, vegetarian, and the other SIBO diets discussed in this book. I hope you enjoy these recipes as you begin your SIBO diet, and that they become an integral part of your healing. Bon appétit!

LEGEND FOR RECIPE LABELS

Bi-Phasic Diet (BPD)

Cedars-Sinai Diet (CSD)

Low-FODMAP (LF)

Low-Histamine (LH)

Specific Carbohydrate Diet (SCD)

SIBO Specific Food Guide (SSFG)

NUTRITIONAL LABELS

Dairy-free

Gluten-free

Nut-free

Vegetarian

Note: Always check ingredient packaging for gluten-free labeling to ensure that foods, especially oats, were processed in a completely gluten-free facility.

Raspberry Orange Muffins, page 61

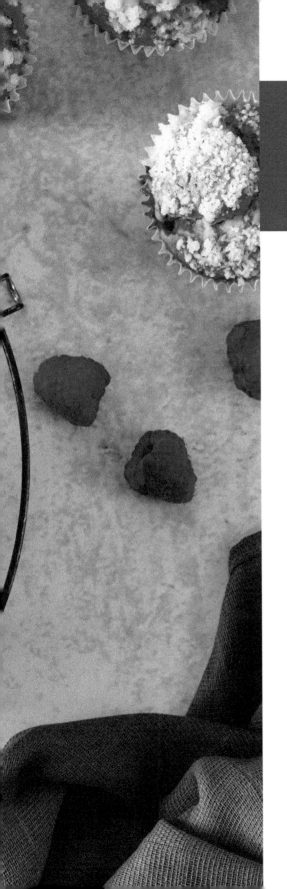

5

Breakfast

Italian Sausage and Egg Scramble

Makes
8
SAUSAGE PATTIES

PREP TIME:
10 MINUTES

COOK TIME:
15 MINUTES

Since commercially made sausages tend to have high-FODMAP ingredients such as garlic, it is best to make your own sausage quickly and easily at home. In this recipe, we combine the sausage with eggs for a delicious morning scramble, but you can also make just the sausage ingredients into patties and cook them separately.

FOR THE SAUSAGE

2 teaspoons Italian herbs (without garlic)

1 teaspoon sea salt

¼ teaspoon freshly ground black pepper

1 tablespoon garlic-infused oil

1 pound ground pork or turkey

FOR THE SCRAMBLE

8 to 12 large eggs (2 per person, depending on how many people you would like to serve)

1 tablespoon unsalted butter or ghee (optional)

Sea salt

Freshly ground black pepper

TO MAKE THE SAUSAGE

1. Put the Italian herbs, salt, pepper, oil, and pork in a medium bowl and mix thoroughly.

2. Put the sausage mixture in a large skillet over medium-high heat and cook while stirring and breaking the meat into smaller pieces. Cook about 10 minutes, or until cooked through.

TO MAKE THE SCRAMBLE

1. Crack the eggs into a medium bowl and whisk them well.

2. Pour the eggs into the skillet with the sausage. Stirring constantly, cook the eggs, 4 to 5 minutes. While the eggs cook, add the butter (if using) and season with salt and pepper to taste. Serve immediately.

▶ **MAKE-AHEAD TIP:** Sausage patties freeze well, so you can make a large batch of these and freeze and defrost them when you need them.

Per serving (2 patties): Calories: 475; Total fat: 37g; Saturated fat: 13g; Cholesterol: 454mg; Sodium: 787mg; Carbohydrates: 1g; Fiber: <1g; Protein: 32g

Sweet Potato Mash

Serves

2

PREP TIME:
10 MINUTES

COOK TIME:
45 MINUTES

This mashed sweet potato recipe is a great addition to any breakfast because it gives you healthy fat from the nut or seed butter, ghee, or oil. It also provides a plentiful, delicious serving of carbs from the sweet potato and honey. Add some protein on the side and you have a tasty, filling breakfast meal to start your day off right. One-half cup of sweet potato is low-FODMAP, so the serving size should be ½ cup or less.

1 medium sweet potato

2 tablespoons ghee, unsalted butter, or coconut oil (use ghee or coconut oil for CSD)

1 teaspoon clover honey (optional)

¼ teaspoon ground cinnamon (optional)

2 tablespoons nut or seed butter (optional)

1. Preheat the oven to 400°F. Line a baking sheet with aluminum foil.

2. Pierce the outside of the sweet potato with a fork and place it on the prepared baking sheet. Bake the sweet potato for about 45 minutes, or until a fork can easily pierce all the way through it.

3. Remove and discard the skin and mash the sweet potato.

4. Mix 1 cup of the mashed sweet potato with the ghee, honey (if using), and cinnamon (if using).

5. Drizzle the sweet potato mixture with the nut butter (if using). Serve immediately.

Per serving: Calories: 203; Total fat: 15g; Saturated fat: 9g; Cholesterol: 30mg; Sodium: 8mg; Carbohydrates: 16g; Fiber: 2g; Protein: 1g

Raspberry Orange Muffins

Serves

12

PREP TIME:
15 MINUTES

COOK TIME:
25 MINUTES

If you are missing the taste of gluten products, especially baked goods like muffins, these raspberry orange muffins taste a lot like the real thing but are low-FODMAP. Instead of traditional flour, which can be irritating for SIBO patients, this recipe uses white rice flour, which is easily digestible but also keeps these muffins tasting delicious. Be sure to use whole cane sugar and not heavily processed white sugar. You can easily make these muffins ahead of time and freeze them for an on-the-go breakfast.

FOR THE STREUSEL TOPPING

- 3 tablespoons whole cane sugar
- 1 tablespoon white rice flour
- 2 teaspoons avocado oil, melted ghee, unsalted butter, or coconut oil (use ghee for CSD)

FOR THE MUFFINS

- 2 cups white rice flour
- 1 tablespoon plus 1 teaspoon baking powder
- 1 teaspoon sea salt
- ¼ cup whole cane sugar
- Grated zest from 1 orange
- 2 large eggs
- 1 cup low-FODMAP milk
- ¼ cup avocado oil
- 1 cup fresh or frozen raspberries

CONTINUED ▶

TO MAKE THE STREUSEL TOPPING

In a small bowl, whisk together the sugar and rice flour. Add the avocado oil and whisk until everything is thoroughly mixed together and it looks slightly pebbly. Set the mixture aside.

TO MAKE THE MUFFINS

1. Preheat the oven to 375°F.

2. Lightly grease a 12-cup muffin tin or silicone muffin pan, or add paper liners to a muffin tin.

3. In a medium bowl, whisk together the rice flour, baking powder, salt, sugar, and orange zest. Make a well in the middle of these dry ingredients.

4. In a small bowl, whisk together the eggs, milk, and oil. Pour this mixture into the well and mix it in with the rest of the dry ingredients until just blended.

5. Gently stir in the raspberries.

6. Scoop the mixture into the prepared muffin cups, filling each about three-fourths full. Sprinkle each muffin with the streusel topping, about 1 teaspoon each. Bake for 20 to 25 minutes, or until the muffins are slightly golden.

7. Cool the muffin tin on a wire rack for 5 minutes before removing the muffins from the tin.

▶ **SIBO TIP:** Most people are able tolerate rice or rice-flour products, but everyone is different, so if you are not sure about your tolerance, taste-test a small amount first.

Per serving (1 muffin): Calories: 202; Total fat: 7g; Saturated fat: 1g; Cholesterol: 31mg; Sodium: 216mg; Carbohydrates: 32g; Fiber: 1g; Protein: 3g

GLUTEN-FREE • NUT-FREE • VEGETARIAN
DIETS: BPD (PHASE 2), LF, SCD, SSFG

Healthy Green Smoothie

Serves

1

PREP TIME:
5 MINUTES

Smoothies are a great way to include healthy fat, protein, and carbohydrates in your diet. Although this healthy green smoothie makes for a well-rounded meal supplement, if you have any food sensitivities or allergies, feel free to leave out or substitute with an ingredient of your choice.

½ **cup low-FODMAP milk**

½ **frozen banana**

¼ **cup blueberries**

1 cup packed spinach leaves

1 teaspoon vanilla extract

2 tablespoons collagen powder or almond butter

1 teaspoon spirulina (optional; do not use for SSFG, BPD, or SCD)

1 teaspoon MCT oil (optional)

1 tablespoon honey or maple syrup (optional; use honey for SCD or maple syrup for low-FODMAP)

Ice cubes (optional)

1. Add the milk, banana, blueberries, spinach, vanilla, collagen, spirulina (if using), MCT oil (if using), and honey (if using) to a blender.

2. Blend for 1 minute, or until smooth.

3. For a thicker or colder smoothie, add 2 ice cubes at a time and blend again until smooth.

▶ **INGREDIENT TIP:** MCT (medium-chain triglyceride) oil provides healthy fat, but some people need to build up a tolerance, as it can cause diarrhea if taken in large doses. I recommend starting with 1 teaspoon and moving up to 1 tablespoon over time.

Per serving: Calories: 200; Total fat: 2g; Saturated fat: <1g; Cholesterol: 1mg; Sodium: 168mg; Carbohydrates: 24g; Fiber: 4g; Protein: 23g

24-Hour Yogurt with Lemon-Berry Compote

Serves

8

PREP TIME:
15 MINUTES

COOK TIME:
**24 HOURS,
PLUS 8 HOURS
CHILLING**

Homemade yogurt is easy and delicious—all it requires is time and an appetite. This recipe for 24-hour yogurt is lactose-free and can become a dietary staple for those who do well with dairy. What really elevates this yogurt recipe is the warm lemon-berry compote, which is also delicious by itself or over pancakes. For SIBO sufferers who tend to be more sensitive to dairy products, try a teaspoon of this yogurt first and then move up to larger amounts as tolerated.

FOR THE YOGURT

15 to 30 ice cubes

Water

2 quarts organic whole milk or half-and-half (or the amount specified on your particular yogurt maker)

1 packet yogurt starter culture

FOR THE LEMON-BERRY COMPOTE

2½ cups fresh or frozen strawberries

¾ cup fresh or frozen raspberries

¾ cup fresh or frozen blueberries

Grated zest of 1 lemon

2 tablespoons ghee, unsalted butter, or coconut oil (use ghee for SCD)

1 tablespoon pasteurized honey, whole cane sugar, or maple syrup (optional)

Cooking thermometer

Yogurt maker (the yogurt can also be made in a slow cooker, an electric pressure cooker, or an oven set to 110°F)

TO MAKE THE YOGURT

1. Fill a large baking pan with the ice cubes and water. Set aside.

2. In a medium saucepan over medium-high heat, heat the milk to about 180°F, using a cooking thermometer to measure the temperature.

3. Set the saucepan in the baking pan among the ice cubes to cool the milk to 110°F.

4. Pour the yogurt starter culture into a separate large bowl or the bowl of a yogurt maker. Add ½ cup of the cooled milk and whisk together until well combined. Add the rest of the milk and mix well. Pour the yogurt mixture into the yogurt maker and cook at 110°F for 24 hours.

5. Remove the yogurt from the machine and chill it for 8 hours, or until it has properly set.

CONTINUED ▶

TO MAKE THE LEMON-BERRY COMPOTE

1. Place the strawberries, raspberries, blueberries, lemon zest, ghee, and honey (if using) in a medium saucepan over medium heat.

2. Bring the fruit mixture to a simmer, stirring occasionally. If it starts to boil or begins to stick to the bottom of the pan, turn down the heat so it just barely simmers.

3. Cook for 15 to 30 minutes, or until the compote begins to thicken. Refrigerate until it cools; then spoon it over the yogurt and serve.

▶ **COOKING TIP:** For a smoother compote, you can purée it with an immersion blender. For a chunkier compote, allow it to cook down and break up the biggest pieces with a wooden spoon as you stir it. I do not typically add sweetener to my compote, but if you want to incorporate extra calories in your diet, adding some is helpful.

Per serving: Calories: 221; Total fat: 12g; Saturated fat: 7g; Cholesterol: 37mg; Sodium: 121mg; Carbohydrates: 21g; Fiber: 2g; Protein: 8g

Warm Cinnamon Rice Cereal

Serves

1 to 2

PREP TIME:

5 MINUTES

COOK TIME:

5 MINUTES

Many people with SIBO tolerate white rice well, which makes this recipe for warm cinnamon rice perfect for an easy, tasty, and soothing breakfast. If you would like, you can mix a large batch of this cereal in advance and have it ready for the week. For a well-rounded meal, you can pair this dish with protein such as eggs or breakfast sausage. If you are making breakfast for your family or friends you can easily double or triple this recipe.

1 cup cooked white rice

⅓ cup low-FODMAP milk

2 teaspoons honey or maple syrup (optional)

¼ teaspoon ground cinnamon (optional)

⅛ cup chopped almonds or walnuts (optional)

⅓ ripe banana, sliced, or ⅓ cup fresh blueberries, raspberries, or sliced strawberries (optional)

In a small saucepan over medium-high heat, add the rice, milk, honey (if using), and cinnamon (if using). Mix thoroughly and stir until warm. Top with nuts or fruit (if using) and serve immediately.

▶ **SIBO TIP:** For a low-histamine diet, use ½ cup of rice, 1 teaspoon honey, just a pinch of cinnamon, and fresh blueberries, raspberries, or strawberries as a topping.

▶ **COOKING TIP:** You can make this recipe even faster by putting the rice, milk, honey, and cinnamon in a microwave-safe bowl and heating the cereal in the microwave for at least 1 minute or until hot.

Per serving: Calories: 231; Total fat: 7g; Saturated fat: <1g; Cholesterol: 0mg; Sodium: 30mg; Carbohydrates: 46g; Fiber: 1g; Protein: 7g

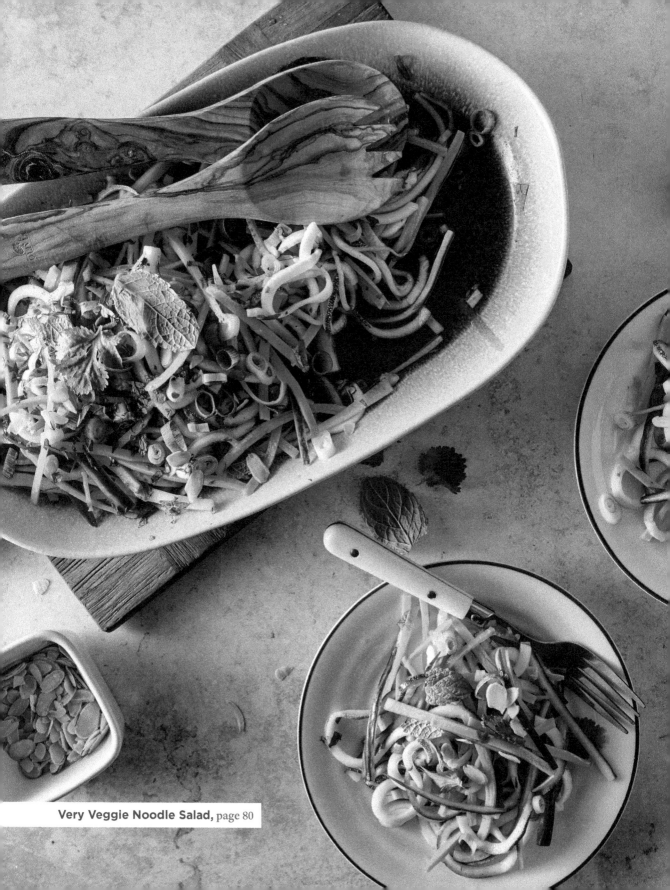

Very Veggie Noodle Salad, page 80

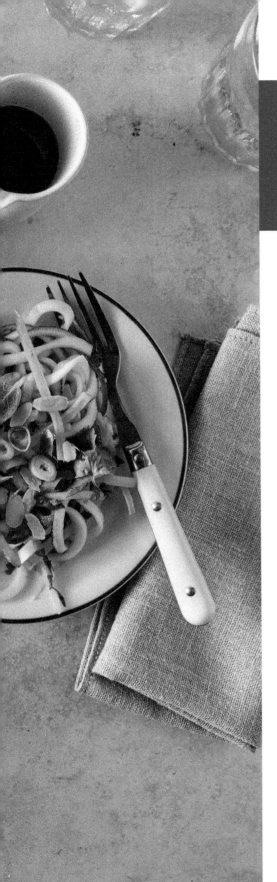

6

Soups, Salads, and Sandwiches

DAIRY-FREE • GLUTEN-FREE • NUT-FREE

DIETS: BPD (PHASE 1), CSD, LF, SCD, SSFG

Low-FODMAP Chicken Bone Broth

Serves

8 to 10

PREP TIME:

10 MINUTES

COOK TIME:

6 HOURS

This broth can be cooked for up to 24 hours, but I find that even 4 to 6 hours of cooking produces a rich, delicious chicken broth. It can be used as an everyday sipping bone broth and as a base for soups or mashed vegetables. It can also be frozen in mason jars or in ice cube trays for smaller amounts. It can be disappointing that it is hard to find SIBO-friendly premade broth but once you taste the difference in this homemade recipe, you will never want to go back!

2 chicken carcasses, meat removed

1 tablespoon apple cider vinegar

1 bunch scallions, coarsely chopped (green parts only)

2 medium carrots, peeled and coarsely chopped

1 celery stalk, coarsely chopped

3 thyme sprigs, tied together, or 2 teaspoons dried thyme

1 bay leaf

1 teaspoon crushed dried green peppercorns or freshly ground black pepper (optional)

Sea salt

1. Put the chicken carcasses in a large soup pot over high heat.

2. Pour enough water into the pot to completely cover the chicken and bring the water to a boil.

3. Reduce the heat to maintain a simmer. Skim off and discard any foam that has risen to the top.

4. Add the vinegar, scallions, carrots, celery, thyme, bay leaf, peppercorns (if using), and salt.

5. Simmer for 4 to 6 hours, adding more water as needed to maintain the original water level.

6. Strain the broth through a fine mesh strainer into a large bowl or other container and let it cool in refrigerator.

7. Transfer the broth to mason jars or glass containers if desired, and refrigerate or freeze. If you are freezing the broth, be sure not to overfill the jars or containers. Consume the refrigerated broth within 3 days.

▶ **SIBO TIP:** Making bone broth with chicken carcasses or other cartilaginous bones will result in a bone broth with GAGs (glycosaminoglycans). GAGs are multichain carbohydrates (polysaccharides) and are generally seen as a beneficial part of bone broth. However, even though they are not high-FODMAP, some people with IBS or SIBO react negatively to them. It is important to test your individual reaction.

Per serving: Calories: 25; Total fat: <1g; Saturated fat: 0g; Cholesterol: 0mg; Sodium: 10mg; Carbohydrates: 5g; Fiber: 1g; Protein: 1g

Crunchy Salad Spring Rolls

Makes
6
WRAPS

PREP TIME:
35 MINUTES

Salad rolls are a great snack, quick lunch, or appetizer. If digesting raw vegetables is difficult for you, blanching or sautéing the harder vegetables (such as carrots) is an option, as well as using more of the other vegetables and leaving out any you do not tolerate. Since white rice is low-FODMAP, many people who have SIBO can easily digest white rice or white-rice products like noodles or wraps. And if you're nonvegetarian and want to punch the recipe up with protein, add in baked chicken.

FOR THE DIPPING SAUCE

- 3 tablespoons rice wine vinegar
- 2 tablespoons olive oil or avocado oil
- 3 tablespoons almond butter or nut butter of choice
- 2 tablespoons coconut aminos
- 1 tablespoon minced peeled fresh ginger

FOR THE SPRING ROLLS

- 6 rice wrappers
- 6 medium to large leaves of soft-leaf lettuce, such as butter lettuce or the soft parts of romaine
- ¾ cup cooked white rice or rice noodles (optional)
- ½ cup thinly sliced, peeled, and seeded cucumber
- ½ cup julienned carrots, blanched or raw
- ¼ cup baby spinach
- ½ cup fresh microgreens
- ½ cup chopped fresh cilantro
- 18 fresh mint leaves
- 1 cup shredded baked chicken (optional)

TO MAKE THE DIPPING SAUCE

In a small bowl, whisk together the vinegar, oil, almond butter, coconut aminos, and ginger. Set aside.

TO MAKE THE SPRING ROLLS

1. Fill a rimmed baking sheet with warm water.

2. Divide the roll ingredients into 6 portions.

3. Place a rice wrapper in the water for 5 to 10 seconds, until it softens; then lay it on a piece of wax or parchment paper or a cutting board.

4. Place a lettuce leaf on the wrapper and then place one portion of each of the rice (if using), cucumber, carrot, spinach, microgreens, cilantro, mint, and chicken (if using) on top of the lettuce in the middle of the wrapper.

5. Fold the sides of the wrapper inward, then roll up the long edge tightly, squeezing the filling to get a tight roll. Repeat for the remaining wrappers.

6. Serve immediately with the dipping sauce or store in the refrigerator.

▶ **PREPARATION TIP:** Learning how to wrap spring rolls can be tricky at first, but several helpful videos are available online. If you have wrapped a burrito before, it is essentially the same technique.

Per serving (1 wrap): Calories: 138; Total fat: 9g; Saturated fat: 1g; Cholesterol: 0mg; Sodium: 134mg; Carbohydrates: 12g; Fiber: 2g; Protein: 3g

Tomato and Cucumber Salad

Serves

4

PREP TIME:
15 MINUTES

Not everyone does well with lettuce at the beginning of a SIBO diet, which can be tricky to navigate when you're craving a salad. This refreshing tomato and cucumber based salad is a great substitute. The cucumbers are peeled and seeded to make them easier to digest, but they still add a nice crunch. This recipe calls for a vinaigrette, but you can substitute Ranch Dressing (see page 159) if desired.

2 cucumbers, peeled, halved, and seeded

1 pint cherry tomatoes, halved

⅛ cup chopped fresh chives or scallions (green parts only)

¼ cup chopped fresh basil (optional)

2 tablespoons olive oil

2 tablespoons garlic-infused oil

2 teaspoons apple cider vinegar

1 teaspoon yellow or Dijon mustard (without garlic)

¼ teaspoon sea salt

⅛ teaspoon freshly ground black pepper

⅓ cup feta cheese or other low-FODMAP cheese aged 30 days or more (optional)

1. Cut the cucumbers into bite-size slices and place them in a medium bowl.

2. Add the tomatoes, chives, and basil (if using) to the bowl with the cucumber slices.

3. Add the olive oil, garlic-infused oil, vinegar, mustard, salt, and pepper to a small mason jar and shake until all the ingredients are thoroughly combined.

4. Pour the dressing over the salad and mix well.

5. Top with the feta cheese (if using). Serve immediately.

▶ **INGREDIENT TIP:** Tomatoes are in the nightshade family and have a reputation for being an inflammatory food. However, scientific research studies paint a different picture. Tomatoes supply bountiful antioxidant and anti-inflammatory phytonutrients that are linked to decreased risk of inflammation and oxidative stress.

Per serving: Calories: 147; Total fat: 14g; Saturated fat: 2g; Cholesterol: 0mg; Sodium: 165mg; Carbohydrates: 5g; Fiber: 2g; Protein: 1g

GLUTEN-FREE • NUT-FREE

DIETS: BPD (PHASE 1), CSD, LF, SCD, SSFG

Carrot Ginger Soup

Serves

8

PREP TIME:
10 MINUTES

COOK TIME:
40 MINUTES

This carrot soup is delicious, satisfying, and warming. For a vegetarian version, use low-FODMAP vegetable broth instead of the chicken broth. I find that using an immersion blender is the best way to purée soups to a smooth and creamy consistency, but if you do not have one, you can use a standard blender to purée the soup in batches. It is very easy to double or triple the batch and freeze some for a week when you do not have time to cook. You can also store the soup in individual jars to grab for a healthy and delicious lunch.

3 tablespoons unsalted butter, ghee, or coconut oil

1 celery stalk, chopped

5 cups chopped carrots or baby carrots

2 tablespoons chopped peeled fresh ginger

6 cups Low-FODMAP Chicken Bone Broth (page 70) or store-bought low-FODMAP vegetable broth

Sea salt

Freshly ground black pepper

1. In a large saucepan, melt the butter over medium-high heat.

2. Add the celery and carrots and cook for 8 minutes, or until the vegetables soften and begin to turn brown. Turn down the heat to medium if needed.

3. Add the ginger and cook for 2 minutes.

4. Pour in the broth and increase the heat to high. Bring the soup to a low boil.

5. Reduce the heat to medium-low and simmer the soup for about 20 minutes, or until the vegetables are tender.

6. Use an immersion blender to purée the soup until it is smooth.

7. Season the soup to taste with salt; if there is no salt in the broth, the soup will need some. Season with pepper to taste, and serve immediately.

▶ **INGREDIENT TIP:** Ginger has been found to be helpful in relieving nausea, dizziness, vomiting, and cold sweats. It also contains anti-inflammatory compounds that may reduce muscular discomfort and pain.

Per serving: Calories: 105; Total fat: 6g; Saturated fat: 3g; Cholesterol: 11mg; Sodium: 70mg; Carbohydrates: 12g; Fiber: 3g; Protein: 2g

Grilled Pesto-Parmesan Sandwich

Serves

1

PREP TIME:
5 MINUTES

COOK TIME:
10 MINUTES

White rice, peeled white potato, and white bread are the three starchier foods I recommend when people are starting a SIBO diet and want or need more carbohydrates. They are helpful staples because they provide necessary calories and are highly glycemic, and therefore easily digestible. They also add variety and a comforting taste to meals. Some people tolerate only one or two of the three options, so it is helpful to test them all. The prosciutto in this sandwich adds a great salty meat element, but it can be left out if you want a vegetarian option or just a yummy grilled-cheese sandwich.

1 teaspoon ghee or avocado oil

1 to 2 pieces prosciutto

1 to 2 tablespoons unsalted butter, ghee, or olive oil

2 slices white sourdough or white gluten-free bread

2 tablespoons Fresh Basil Pesto (page 157)

⅓ cup freshly shredded Parmesan cheese (optional)

1. Heat the ghee in a sauté pan or skillet over medium heat.

2. Cook the prosciutto for 2 to 3 minutes, or until each side turns light brown.

3. Remove from the heat and set aside.

4. Using a knife or a pastry brush, spread the butter on the outside of both bread slices.

5. Spread the pesto on the inside of both bread slices.

6. Put the pan that was used for the prosciutto back over medium heat.

7. Place one of the bread slices into the pan, butter-side down and pesto-side up.

8. Sprinkle the cheese over the pesto and top with the prosciutto.

9. Lay the second bread slice on top of the prosciutto, butter-side up.

10. Cook for 1 to 3 minutes on each side, pressing the sandwich with a spatula and flipping it when the first side has turned golden brown.

11. Remove the sandwich from the heat when the cheese has melted, and serve immediately.

▶ **INGREDIENT TIP:** This sandwich can easily be made gluten-free by using a gluten-free white bread in place of the sourdough. I recommend that people get a celiac test before they exclude gluten from their diet. If they already have a negative celiac test, I still recommend eliminating gluten for 4 to 6 weeks. If you have already done an elimination diet and do not react to gluten, I recommend sourdough bread, as the fermentation process lowers the amount of gluten. For those eating gluten-free bread, check to see if you tolerate it, as it is typically made from a mix of flours and contains gums. If you have not been eating bread, I recommend first testing your reaction to a piece of toast by itself before trying this delicious sandwich.

Per serving: Calories: 692; Total fat: 51g; Saturated fat: 17g; Cholesterol: 63mg; Sodium: 1,318mg; Carbohydrates: 45g; Fiber: 2g; Protein: 14g

DAIRY-FREE • GLUTEN-FREE
DIETS: BPD (PHASE 2), CSD, LF, SCD, SSFG

Very Veggie Noodle Salad

Serves

4 to 6

PREP TIME:
15 MINUTES

The colorful vegetables that serve as the noodles in this recipe make for a really beautiful salad. If you do not own a spiralizer yet, I highly recommend it! Spiralized vegetables are a great way to get make easy veggie "pasta" and you can pick up a spiralizer online for under $10. If a spiralizer is not for you or is not available, feel free to slice the vegetables thinly with a knife or a mandoline to create a noodlelike look and feel. With the fish sauce, check the ingredients on the label to make sure the sauce is made with only anchovies and salt; most brands add other ingredients. Leave out the chopped almonds to make this dish nut-free.

¼ cup rice vinegar (without added sugar)

2 tablespoons freshly squeezed lime juice

2 teaspoons fish sauce

1 tablespoon whole cane sugar (substitute honey for BPD, SCD, or SSFG)

½ teaspoon low-FODMAP hot sauce (optional)

1 large English cucumber

1 small zucchini

2 medium carrots

1 bunch fresh cilantro, chopped

1 bunch fresh mint, chopped

4 scallions, chopped (green parts only)

½ cup chopped roasted almonds (optional)

1. In a large bowl, whisk together the vinegar, lime juice, fish sauce, sugar, and hot sauce (if using). Set aside.

2. Peel and spiralize the cucumber and zucchini.

3. Peel and spiralize, shred, or julienne the carrots.

4. In a large bowl, combine the cucumber, zucchini, carrots, cilantro, and mint.

5. Add the vinegar mixture and toss to coat the vegetables.

6. Top with the scallions and almonds (if using). Serve immediately.

▶ **SUBSTITUTION TIP:** This vegetable noodle salad uses a traditional Vietnamese dressing, but if you do not like or cannot obtain fish sauce, you can always substitute Ranch Dressing (see page 159) or a vinaigrette.

Per serving: Calories: 59; Total fat: <1g; Saturated fat: 0g; Cholesterol: 0mg; Sodium: 259mg; Carbohydrates: 13g; Fiber: 5g; Protein: 2g

Sesame Ginger Bok Choy, page 88

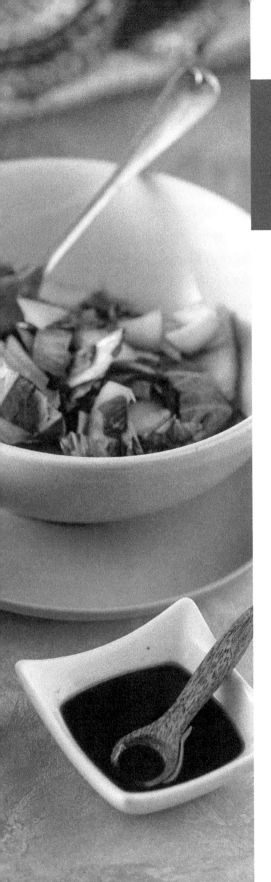

7

Side Dishes

GLUTEN-FREE • NUT-FREE • VEGETARIAN
DIETS: CSD, LF, SCD, SSFG

Orange Carrot Purée

Serves

4

PREP TIME:
5 MINUTES

COOK TIME:
25 MINUTES

This carrot purée is slightly sweet and can be enjoyed for breakfast, lunch, or dinner. If you like and tolerate them, other spices like cinnamon, cumin, or curry can be added to give more depth to the purée. This smooth carrot side dish pairs well with most meats and fish. If you enjoy and can handle spicier food, it works very well with a dash of cayenne or red pepper flakes for some heat. You can store this carrot purée in the refrigerator for up to 1 week.

1 pound carrots, peeled and coarsely chopped

2 tablespoons unsalted butter, ghee, or coconut oil

Grated zest of 1 orange

2 tablespoons freshly squeezed orange juice

¼ teaspoon sea salt, plus more to taste

Freshly ground black pepper

1. Steam the carrots for about 20 minutes, or until they are very soft.

2. Place the carrots in a food processor or blender and add the butter, orange zest, orange juice, and salt.

3. Process for 1 minute, or until all the ingredients are puréed together.

4. Taste and add more salt and pepper as desired. Serve immediately.

▶ **SIBO TIP:** Puréed vegetables are an important part of starting a SIBO diet because they are easy to digest. Carrots are naturally easy to steam and purée, and their flavor can be switched up by pairing them with different spices and herbs.

Per serving: Calories: 102; Total fat: 6g; Saturated fat: 4g; Cholesterol: 15mg; Sodium: 224mg; Carbohydrates: 12g; Fiber: 3g; Protein: 1g

Sautéed Fennel and Radishes with Chives

Serves

2

PREP TIME:
5 MINUTES

COOK TIME:
5 MINUTES

Most people think of eating radishes raw, but cooking them gives them a little softness, in both taste and texture. Sautéing the fennel and radishes together caramelizes them a bit, enriching their flavor. They may be vegetables you do not eat too often, but it is very important to keep your diet as diverse as possible which makes this dish perfect for supporting your microbiome.

1 tablespoon ghee, unsalted butter, or olive oil

1 bunch radishes, trimmed and quartered

1 cup chopped cored fennel

Sea salt

Freshly ground black pepper

1 tablespoon chopped chives

1. In a sauté pan or skillet, heat the ghee over medium heat until it melts and begins to sizzle lightly.

2. Add the radishes and fennel to the pan. Sauté the vegetables for 5 minutes, or until they turn golden brown but are not burnt, reducing the heat as needed.

3. Remove from the heat.

4. Add salt and pepper to taste and sprinkle the chives over the top. Serve immediately.

▶ **INGREDIENT TIP:** Fennel is a member of the carrot family and contains phytonutrients that give it strong antioxidant properties. Note that you will want to cut out its tough core before slicing the rest of it.

Per serving: Calories: 74; Total fat: 6g; Saturated fat: 4g; Cholesterol: 15mg; Sodium: 46mg; Carbohydrates: 5g; Fiber: 2g; Protein: 1g

GLUTEN-FREE · NUT-FREE · VEGETARIAN
DIETS: BPD (PHASE 2), LF, SCD, SSFG

Parmesan Crisps

Makes
24
CRISPS

PREP TIME:
5 MINUTES

COOK TIME:
15 MINUTES

Aged cheese can be a very supportive part of a SIBO diet, as the fat in cheese is satiating and will tide you over until the next meal. These crisps are delicious as a snack, or as a topping for soups or salads. Make these ahead and store in an airtight container or storage bag in the refrigerator for easy snacking. Making Parmesan crisps yourself is much more cost-effective than buying them at the supermarket.

1 cup freshly and finely grated Parmesan cheese (aged 30 days or more)

1. Preheat the oven to 400°F. Line two baking sheets with silicone baking mats or parchment paper.

2. Using a heaping tablespoon for each round, make 12 small rounds of Parmesan on each sheet, evenly spacing them in four rows of three across.

3. Place the first baking sheet in the oven and bake for 5 to 7 minutes. The crisps should look lacy and golden but not brown.

4. Remove the sheet from the oven and place it on a wire rack to cool.

5. Repeat with the second sheet.

6. When the crisps are cool, remove them from the baking sheets and serve them immediately.

▶ **INGREDIENT TIP:** You can try this recipe with any other low-FODMAP cheese. Keep an eye on them because baking times may differ slightly with different cheeses.

Per serving (1 crisp): Calories: 22; Total fat: 2g; Saturated fat: 1g; Cholesterol: 5mg; Sodium: 83mg; Carbohydrates: 0g; Fiber: 0g; Protein: 2g

Sautéed Lemon Spinach

Serves

4

PREP TIME:
3 MINUTES

COOK TIME:
10 MINUTES

Spinach, for those who tolerate it well, is a great green to sauté on a SIBO-centric diet because it becomes soft and cooking makes it easier to digest. Make sure to buy organic spinach, as it is one of the Dirty Dozen™ produce that contains the most pesticide residue if farmed conventionally.

1 teaspoon ghee or unsalted butter (use ghee for SCD)

2 teaspoons garlic-infused oil

Grated zest of 1 organic lemon

4 cups organic spinach, packed

2 teaspoons freshly squeezed lemon juice

Sea salt

Freshly ground black pepper

1. In a large skillet, heat the ghee and oil over medium heat until they melt and combine.

2. Add the lemon zest and spinach to the ghee and oil mixture and sauté until the spinach wilts, about 3 minutes.

3. Remove from the heat and add the lemon juice, plus salt and pepper to taste. Serve immediately.

▶ **INGREDIENT TIP:** Add chopped spinach to soups or stews when you can, as it is an excellent source of vitamins A, E, B_2, B_6, and K, iron, magnesium, manganese, and folate.

Per serving: Calories: 39; Total fat: 4g; Saturated fat: 1g; Cholesterol: 3mg; Sodium: 30mg; Carbohydrates: 2g; Fiber: 1g; Protein: 1g

Sesame Ginger Bok Choy

Serves

4

PREP TIME:
10 MINUTES

COOK TIME:
10 MINUTES

Bok choy may seem like an uncommon vegetable to add to your diet, but it is a great way to add variety to your SIBO diet. Additionally, bok choy is an excellent source of vitamins A and C and manganese. It can be sautéed by itself in oil, but here we add Asian-inspired flavors to kick this side dish up a notch. The ginger in this recipe is a great addition because the root is known for its anti-inflammatory properties as well as its ability to reduce motion sickness.

1 pound baby bok choy

1½ tablespoons coconut aminos

1 tablespoon rice vinegar (without added sugar)

¼ teaspoon whole cane sugar (substitute honey for BPD and SSFG)

1 tablespoon avocado oil

1 garlic clove

1 tablespoon finely chopped peeled fresh ginger

2 teaspoons sesame oil

1. Cut off the main stem of the bok choy and rinse the leaves separately to remove any dirt. Chop the leaves into bite-size pieces.

2. Put the coconut aminos, vinegar, and sugar in a small bowl and whisk together. Set aside.

3. Heat a large skillet over medium-high heat. Add the avocado oil and swirl it to coat the bottom of the pan.

4. Add the garlic and ginger to the pan and sauté for 1 minute, or until they become fragrant. Remove the garlic and discard it.

5. Put the bok choy in the pan and sauté for about 3 minutes, or until it is tender.

6. Add the amino mixture and sauté for 1 more minute.

7. Remove the pan from the heat and add the sesame oil, stirring to mix. Serve immediately.

▶ **SIBO TIP:** This recipe uses a garlic clove to flavor the oil but then discards it, making the dish low-FODMAP but still giving you that beautiful garlic smell and taste.

Per serving: Calories: 86; Total fat: 6g; Saturated fat: 1g; Cholesterol: 0mg; Sodium: 226mg; Carbohydrates: 7g; Fiber: 1g; Protein: 1g

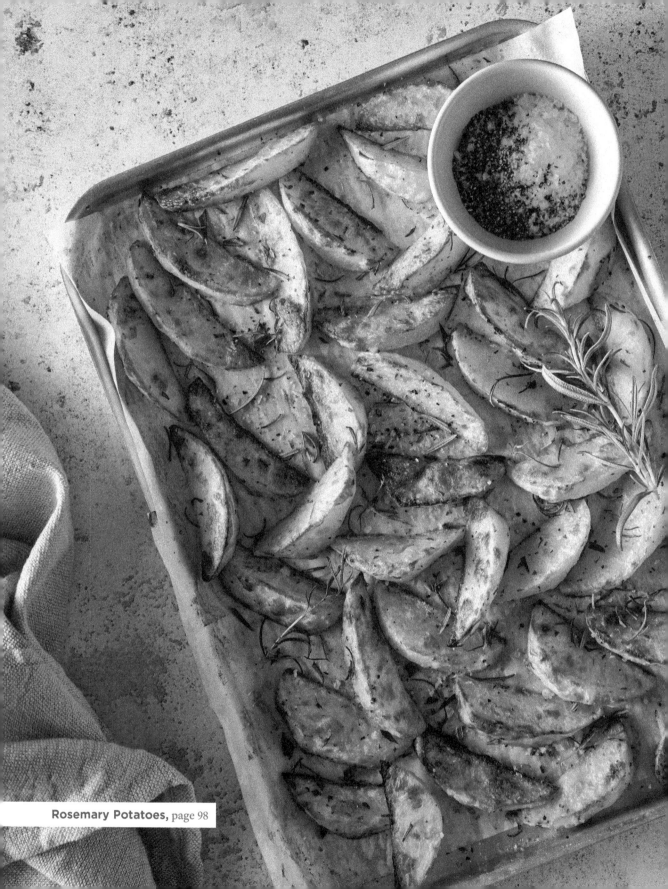

Rosemary Potatoes, page 98

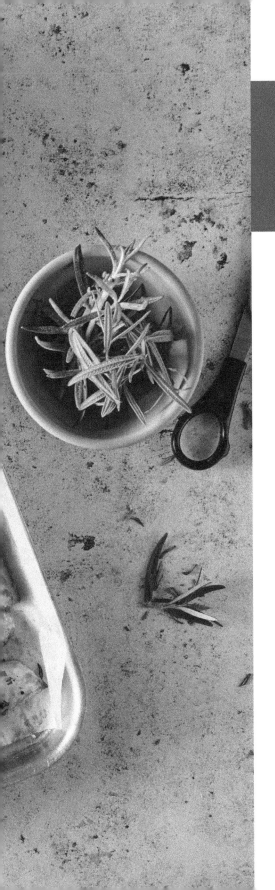

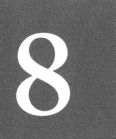

8

Rice and Potatoes

Easy Fried Rice

Serves

6

PREP TIME:
15 MINUTES

COOK TIME:
15 MINUTES

Fried rice can be such a treat, especially when eating out. Most restaurants use soy, gluten, MSG, and other ingredients that might not work on a SIBO diet. But this fried rice is easy to make and enjoy at home. You can eat it alone as an entrée, as a side, or paired with the Teriyaki Chicken Skewers (see page 106).

1 egg yolk

3 cups cooked and cooled white rice

3 tablespoons unsalted butter, ghee, or avocado oil (use ghee or avocado oil for CSD), divided

2 large eggs

2 medium carrots, peeled and diced

20 snow peas, sliced

4 scallions, sliced (green parts only)

¼ cup coconut aminos

1 teaspoon sesame oil

1. In a bowl, mix the egg yolk into the rice until the rice is coated. Set aside.

2. In a large sauté pan or skillet, heat 1 tablespoon of the butter over medium heat.

3. Crack the eggs into a small bowl and whisk to combine the yolks and whites. Add the eggs to the pan and stir until cooked, 4 to 5 minutes. Remove the scrambled eggs from the pan and set aside.

4. Put another tablespoon of butter in the pan and add the carrots and snow peas.

5. Sauté the vegetables for about 4 minutes, or until the carrots turn soft. Adjust the heat as needed.

6. Add the remaining tablespoon of butter to the vegetables in the pan and let it melt.

7. Add the rice mixture, scallions, and coconut aminos and stir until well combined. Continue to stir and cook for about 5 minutes.

8. Put the scrambled egg back into the pan and stir to combine. Remove from the heat and stir in the sesame oil.

9. Serve immediately or store in the refrigerator for up to 3 days.

▶ INGREDIENT TIP: You can vary the vegetables in this recipe to use whatever you have on hand. Just make sure to change the cooking time as needed. You can also add more coconut aminos or a little bit of salt to taste.

Per serving: Calories: 236; Total fat: 9g; Saturated fat: 4g; Cholesterol: 108mg; Sodium: 266mg; Carbohydrates: 32g; Fiber: 1g; Protein: 5g

Simple Spanish-Style Fried Rice

Serves

4 to 6

PREP TIME:
10 MINUTES

COOK TIME:
25 MINUTES

This Spanish-style rice is easy to make, and you can always double the recipe for a big event or to save for later. When starting a SIBO diet, it can be exciting to look for recipes that mixed things up so you don't feel as if you are eating the same old dishes over and over. If you need to leave out certain vegetables, like the scallions or the bell pepper, it will not have a major effect on the recipe. To make this vegetarian, use low-FODMAP vegetable broth instead of chicken broth.

2 tablespoons avocado oil

3 scallions, sliced (green parts only)

1½ cups uncooked long-grain white rice

1 red bell pepper, diced

2 cups Low-FODMAP Chicken Bone Broth (page 70) or store-bought low-FODMAP vegetable broth

1 cup diced tomatoes, with juice

1 tablespoon freshly squeezed lemon juice

½ teaspoon ground cumin

½ teaspoon chili powder (optional)

1 teaspoon sea salt

1 tablespoon garlic-infused oil

1. In a large saucepan, heat the avocado oil over medium heat and swirl to coat the pan.

2. Put the scallions in the pan and sauté until tender, about 2 minutes.

3. Add the rice to the pan and continue to cook. When the rice begins to turn golden brown, add the bell pepper, broth, tomatoes with their juices, lemon juice, cumin, chili powder (if using), salt, and garlic-infused oil.

4. Reduce the heat, cover, and simmer for about 20 minutes, or until the liquid is absorbed. Serve immediately.

▶ **INGREDIENT NOTE:** To lower the levels of arsenic in rice, the Environmental Working Group recommends soaking the rice overnight in water before cooking, cooking the rice in the excess soaking liquid, and then draining off the extra liquid. White jasmine or basmati rice from California or Southeast Asia tends to have lower concentrations of arsenic. In this recipe, we do not cook the rice in the excess liquid, but you can soak it before using it.

Per serving: Calories: 382; Total fat: 11g; Saturated fat: 2g; Cholesterol: 0mg; Sodium: 596mg; Carbohydrates: 63g; Fiber: 3g; Protein: 6g

DAIRY-FREE · GLUTEN-FREE · NUT-FREE · VEGETARIAN
DIETS: BPD (PHASE 2), CSD, LF

French Potato Salad

Serves

8

PREP TIME:
10 MINUTES

COOK TIME:
30 MINUTES

A French potato salad uses vinaigrette as the dressing instead of a mayonnaise base. I suggest that you serve the salad warm, but it is also tasty at room temperature. Since this serves eight, it makes a great salad to take to a picnic or a fun barbecue. You can also halve the recipe if you want a smaller amount.

1½ teaspoons sea salt, divided

2 pounds medium red or white boiling potatoes

¼ cup olive oil

¼ cup garlic-infused oil

1½ tablespoons red wine vinegar

1½ tablespoons freshly squeezed lemon juice

1 tablespoon Dijon or yellow mustard (without garlic)

¼ teaspoon freshly ground black pepper

¼ cup chopped scallions (green parts only)

2 tablespoons minced fresh dill

2 tablespoons minced fresh flat-leaf parsley

1. Fill a large pot with water, add 1 teaspoon of the salt, and warm it over high heat.

2. Peel the potatoes, cut them into large chunks (about 8 pieces per potato), and drop them into the salted water.

3. Cook the potatoes for 20 to 30 minutes, until they are just cooked through but not mushy. Remove them from the heat and drain them in a colander.

4. While the potatoes cook, make the vinaigrette. Combine the olive oil, garlic-infused oil, vinegar, lemon juice, mustard, the remaining ½ teaspoon salt, and pepper in a mason jar and shake until all the ingredients are well combined.

5. Place the potatoes in a medium bowl. Add the vinaigrette, scallions, dill, and parsley and mix everything well. Serve warm or at room temperature.

▶ **VARIATION TIP:** This potato salad is delicious on its own, but to make it into a more robust meal, add halved cherry tomatoes, quartered hardboiled eggs, halved olives, steamed green beans or haricots verts, and tuna or chicken.

Per serving: Calories: 203; Total fat: 14g; Saturated fat: 2g; Cholesterol: 0mg; Sodium: 503mg; Carbohydrates: 19g; Fiber: 2g; Protein: 2g

Rosemary Potatoes

Serves

4 to 6

PREP TIME:
10 MINUTES

COOK TIME:
40 MINUTES

Rosemary potatoes are a delicious side dish for breakfast or dinner. These go extremely well with Citrus Chicken with Olives and Artichoke Hearts (see page 108). Potatoes are high-glycemic (so they have low fermentation potential) and contain a small amount of fiber without their skins, so many people tolerate them if they do well with starchier vegetables.

1½ pounds medium red- or white-skinned potatoes, peeled and cut into bite-size chunks

2 tablespoons olive oil

1 tablespoon garlic-infused oil

2 tablespoons finely chopped fresh rosemary leaves

½ teaspoon freshly ground black pepper (optional; remove for the Low-Histamine diet)

1 teaspoon sea salt

1. Preheat the oven to 400°F. Line a baking sheet with parchment paper or aluminum foil.

2. Place the potatoes on the prepared baking sheet and add the olive oil, garlic-infused oil, rosemary, pepper (if using), and salt.

3. Mix the ingredients together with your hands or a wooden spoon, and then spread them out evenly on the baking sheet.

4. Place the baking sheet in the oven and bake for 20 minutes.

5. Flip the potatoes with a spatula so they brown evenly.

6. Bake for another 20 minutes, or until the potatoes are golden brown and cooked through. Serve immediately.

▶ **SIBO TIP:** If you do well with a little bit of fiber, you can leave the potato skin on, but I highly recommend that people who are symptomatic peel all their vegetables when starting a SIBO-friendly diet.

Per serving: Calories: 210; Total fat: 11g; Saturated fat: 1g; Cholesterol: 0mg; Sodium: 612mg; Carbohydrates: 27g; Fiber: 3g; Protein: 3g

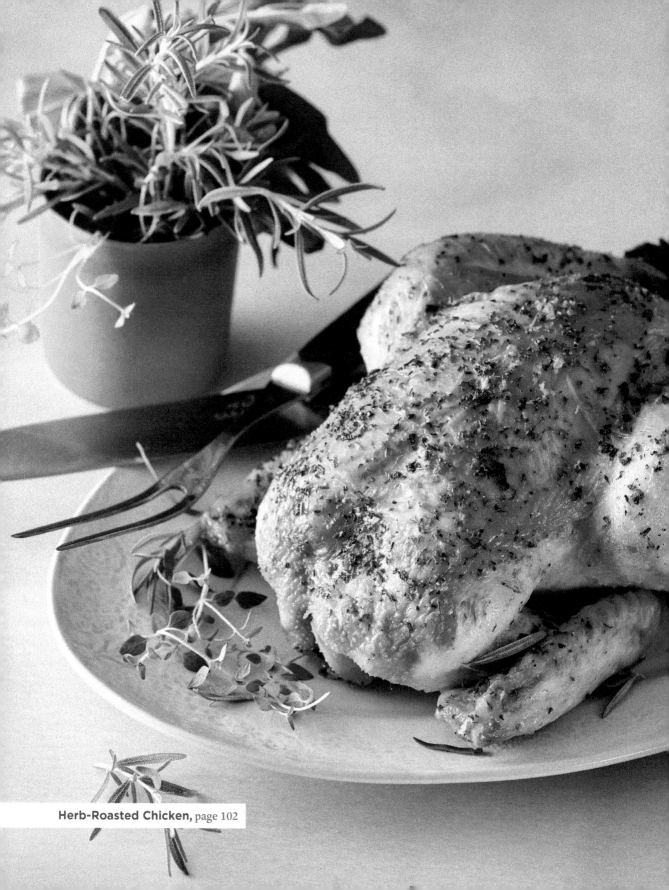

Herb-Roasted Chicken, page 102

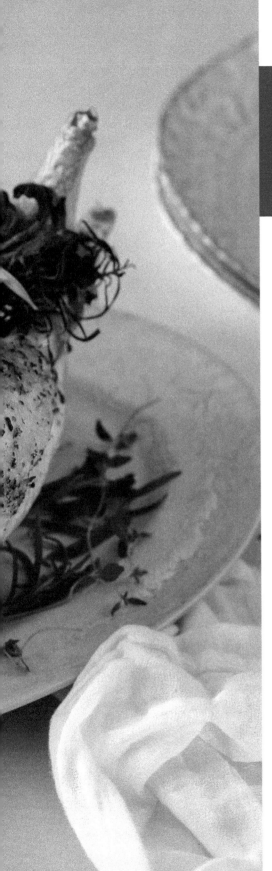

Poultry

DAIRY-FREE • GLUTEN-FREE • NUT-FREE
DIETS: BPD (PHASE 1), CSD, LF, LH (PHASE 1), SCD, SSFG

Herb-Roasted Chicken

Serves

4 to 6

PREP TIME:
5 MINUTES

COOK TIME:
1 HOUR
40 MINUTES

Roasting a chicken is such an easy thing to do once you get the hang of it. It is lovely to smell it cooking, see its golden color as you take it out of the oven, and maybe steal a piece of crispy skin while you wait for it to cool. It is also helpful to cook a chicken on the weekend to use in other dishes throughout the week. Food prepping can be fun and delicious! If you want to truss your chicken (tie string around it to keep the wings and legs close to the body to help it cook evenly), make sure to look online for step-by-step instructions and use kitchen twine.

1 (5- to 6-pound) whole chicken

3 or 4 fresh or dried herb sprigs, such as thyme, sage, or rosemary

1 tablespoon melted coconut oil, unsalted butter, or ghee (use ghee for CSD)

1 teaspoon dried Italian seasoning (without garlic) or herbes de Provence

Sea salt

Freshly ground black pepper (optional; remove for the Low-Histamine diet)

1. Preheat the oven to 400°F. Line a baking sheet with parchment paper or aluminum foil.

2. Pat the chicken until it is dry, and place it on the baking sheet.

3. Place the herb sprigs inside the chicken cavity and truss the chicken if desired.

4. Using a pastry brush, brush the chicken with the coconut oil.

5. Generously sprinkle the chicken with the Italian seasoning, salt, and pepper (if using).

6. Roast for 90 minutes, or until the chicken is fully cooked and its juices run clear. If you use a meat thermometer, insert it into the thickest part of the thigh without touching the bone. The temperature should be at least 165°F.

7. Remove the chicken from the oven and let it rest for 10 minutes before cutting and serving.

▶ **SIBO TIP:** During Phase 1 of the Low-Histamine and Bi-Phasic diets, do not eat the chicken skin. During Phase 2, the skin can be consumed.

Per serving (¼ of chicken): Calories: 326; Total fat: 11g; Saturated fat: 6g; Cholesterol: 172mg; Sodium: 190mg; Carbohydrates: <1g; Fiber: <1g; Protein: 52g

Five-Spice Baked Chicken Wings with Sesame Dipping Sauce

Serves

4

PREP TIME:
10 MINUTES

COOK TIME:
40 MINUTES

These chicken wings get deliciously crispy in the oven. While they are incredibly flavorful by themselves, with the five spices, you can add the sesame dipping sauce for an extra-tasty kick. These wings can be part of an easy weeknight meal paired with Sesame Ginger Bok Choy (see page 88), or they make a great appetizer to take to a party.

2 pounds chicken wings

1 tablespoon gluten-free baking powder

¾ teaspoon sea salt

1 teaspoon five-spice powder

¼ teaspoon freshly ground white pepper

¼ cup coconut aminos

1½ teaspoons rice vinegar (without added sugar)

1 teaspoon sesame oil

1 teaspoon garlic-infused oil

1 teaspoon honey

1. Preheat the oven to 400°F. Line a baking sheet with parchment paper or aluminum foil.

2. Thoroughly pat the chicken wings dry. In a small bowl, mix the baking powder, salt, five-spice powder, and pepper.

3. Dredge the wings in the powder mixture and toss until they are thoroughly coated and the spice mixture is used up.

4. Place the wings on the prepared baking sheet and bake for 30 to 40 minutes, or until they are cooked through.

5. While the wings are cooking, put the coconut aminos, vinegar, sesame oil, garlic-infused oil, and honey in a small bowl and whisk thoroughly. Pour the sauce into an appropriate bowl for dipping and serve immediately with the chicken when it is done.

▶ **SIBO TIP:** Because of the amount of skin on chicken wings, they contain added fat, which can be helpful to add calories to the diet of someone with unwanted weight loss. However, those with fat malabsorption may not tolerate much chicken skin. Start with a small amount to see how you do.

Per serving: Calories: 484; Total fat: 36g; Saturated fat: 10g; Cholesterol: 210mg; Sodium: 1,158mg; Carbohydrates: 6g; Fiber: <1g; Protein: 34g

Teriyaki Chicken Skewers

Serves

4

PREP TIME:
25 MINUTES,
PLUS 8
HOURS TO
MARINATE

COOK TIME:
15 MINUTES

These skewers are great to prep the night before so they are ready to cook for dinner the next evening. They are an especially delicious companion to Easy Fried Rice (see page 92). You can also cut up the cooked marinated chicken and use it in a chicken salad or a variety of other dishes. These skewers are always a big hit at barbecues and potlucks so feel free to make them often and share them!

FOR THE MARINADE

¼ cup coconut aminos

1 tablespoon honey

1 teaspoon apple
    cider vinegar

1 tablespoon grated
    peeled fresh ginger

1 teaspoon garlic-infused oil

FOR THE CHICKEN

1 pound boneless and
    skinless chicken thighs

1 tablespoon avocado oil

FOR THE MARINADE

In a medium bowl, combine the coconut aminos, honey, vinegar, ginger, and garlic-infused oil. Set aside.

FOR THE CHICKEN

1. Cut each chicken thigh in half lengthwise.
2. Add the chicken to the bowl of marinade and stir to coat each piece thoroughly.

3. Cover the chicken and marinade with plastic wrap and marinate overnight.

4. Before cooking the chicken, soak wooden skewers in water for 20 minutes to prevent the wood from splitting or burning.

5. Remove the chicken from the marinade and pat dry.

6. Thread each piece of chicken thigh onto the skewers.

7. Preheat an outdoor grill or indoor grill pan over medium heat. Brush the grill or pan with the avocado oil.

8. Grill the chicken skewers for about 15 minutes, turning as needed, until they are golden brown on both sides and cooked through. Serve immediately.

▶ **EQUIPMENT TIP:** If you do not have wooden skewers, you can cook the thighs directly on the barbecue or a grill pan for the same flavor.

Per serving: Calories: 205; Total fat: 12g; Saturated fat: 3g; Cholesterol: 90mg; Sodium: 499mg; Carbohydrates: 8g; Fiber: 0g; Protein: 16g

Citrus Chicken with Olives and Artichoke Hearts

Serves

4 to 6

PREP TIME:
15 MINUTES

COOK TIME:
35 MINUTES

The capers, kalamata olives, and artichokes give this chicken dish a delicious Mediterranean taste. I love to use fresh herbs in recipes whenever I can since they have a bright flavor and wonderful smell and they can really change the taste of a dish. Whether you live in a house or an apartment, or consider yourself to have a green thumb, growing an herb garden is easy with a sunny window. I recommend thyme, chives, basil, and parsley to make the most of your everyday dishes.

6 bone-in, skin-on chicken thighs

Sea salt

Freshly ground black pepper

2 tablespoons avocado oil

1 tablespoon chopped fresh rosemary

1 lemon, quartered

1 orange, quartered

½ cup pitted kalamata olives

½ cup pitted Castelvetrano olives

2 tablespoons drained capers

1 (14-ounce) can quartered artichoke hearts, drained

½ cup Low-FODMAP Chicken Bone Broth (page 70) or store-bought low-FODMAP chicken broth

2 tablespoons chopped fresh parsley

1. Pat the chicken dry and season it generously with salt and pepper.

2. In a large cast iron skillet or saucepan over medium heat, heat the avocado oil until it is hot but not smoking.

3. Place the chicken skin-side down into the oil and cook for 12 to 14 minutes, or until it is well browned.

4. Remove the chicken and place the pieces skin-side up on a plate. Set aside.

5. Put the rosemary, lemon wedges, orange wedges, kalamata and Castelvetrano olives, capers, artichoke hearts, and chicken broth in the same skillet. Bring to a boil over medium-high heat.

6. Nestle the chicken pieces back into the mixture, lower the heat to medium, cover, and cook for another 15 minutes, or until the chicken is cooked through.

7. Remove the citrus pieces and divide the chicken and olive mixture among serving plates. Serve immediately.

▶ INGREDIENT TIP: Globe artichokes are high-FODMAP, but a half-cup serving of canned artichoke hearts is low-FODMAP because the FODMAPs leach from the artichokes into the canning liquid. I am not usually a huge proponent of canned vegetables, but in this case it works: You can try a vegetable you might otherwise not be able to eat often, and using these canned hearts is much easier than preparing fresh artichokes.

Per serving: Calories: 557; Total fat: 40g; Saturated fat: 9g; Cholesterol: 142mg; Sodium: 668mg; Carbohydrates: 17g; Fiber: 8g; Protein: 31g

Sage Parmesan Meatballs

Makes
24
MEATBALLS

PREP TIME:
10 MINUTES

COOK TIME:
20 MINUTES

Sage and Parmesan cheese are a classic Italian combination that makes these meatballs a hit! These meatballs are delicious by themselves, with a red sauce, with my Fresh Basil Pesto (see page 157), over vegetables, or on low-FODMAP pasta. The recipe can be doubled or tripled, and the meatballs can be frozen and reheated. You can use pork, turkey, chicken, or even a combination of ground meats. As you can see, this recipe is very versatile, and I love using it as a base for adding new flavors to meals. Note that if you are on the SCD or SSFG diet, use only pork rinds made without added garlic or onion.

1 pound ground turkey, chicken, or pork

½ cup cooked white rice or low-FODMAP pork rinds, ground

1 large egg, beaten

1 tablespoon garlic-infused oil

¼ cup finely chopped scallions (green parts only)

1 cup finely shredded Parmesan cheese

2 tablespoons chopped fresh sage

2 tablespoons finely chopped fresh parsley

1 teaspoon sea salt

½ teaspoon freshly ground black pepper

1. Preheat the oven to 400°F. Line a baking sheet with parchment paper or aluminum foil.

2. Combine the ground turkey, rice, egg, oil, scallions, cheese, sage, parsley, salt, and pepper in a large bowl and mix thoroughly.

3. Form the mixture into 1½-inch balls and place them on the baking sheet.

4. Bake for 20 minutes, or until cooked through.

▶ INGREDIENT TIP: We use egg and white rice or pork rinds as binders in this recipe to hold the meatballs together. However, you can swap the egg with a tolerated egg replacer (like gelatin, flax, or chia seeds) and replace the rice or ground pork rinds with sourdough or gluten-free bread crumbs as tolerated.

Per serving (6 meatballs): Calories: 344; Total fat: 20g; Saturated fat: 7g; Cholesterol: 146mg; Sodium: 1,065mg; Carbohydrates: 9g; Fiber: 2g; Protein: 33g

Tender Poached Chicken Breasts

Serves

2 to 4

PREP TIME:
5 MINUTES

COOK TIME:
25 MINUTES

Poached chicken breasts are easy to make and great to have around. If you are having a flare and trying to eat simple meals for a couple of days, it is helpful to eat just the chicken on its own. Poached chicken is also easy to add to other off-the-cuff dishes, such as a chicken salad or vegetable-and-chicken stir-fry, or even just serve over rice or pasta.

2 chicken breasts

1 thyme sprig

1 sage sprig

1 rosemary sprig

1 bay leaf

3 to 4 cups Low-FODMAP Chicken Bone Broth (page 70), store-bought low-FODMAP vegetable broth, or water

1. Place the chicken breasts, thyme, sage, rosemary, and bay leaf in a medium saucepan.

2. Pour the broth over the chicken and herbs. Most of the chicken should be covered with liquid.

3. Bring the mixture to a simmer over medium heat and then turn the heat down to low.

4. Cook the chicken, uncovered, for about 15 minutes.

5. Use a meat thermometer to ensure the internal temperature of the chicken is at least 165°F. If it is not, continue to cook.

6. Once the temperature reaches 165°F, remove the chicken from the poaching liquid.

7. Allow the chicken to cool. When it is cool enough to touch, slice it and serve immediately with some of the poaching liquid over it, or refrigerate it until you are ready to use it.

▶ **COOKING TIP:** If you do not have the herbs listed in this recipe on hand or if you want to try a different twist, use peppercorns, lemon juice, five-spice powder, or your own preferred herbs, citrus, or spices to flavor the water or broth.

Per serving: Calories: 150; Total fat: 3g; Saturated fat: 1g; Cholesterol: 65mg; Sodium: 195mg; Carbohydrates: 8g; Fiber: 2g; Protein: 25g

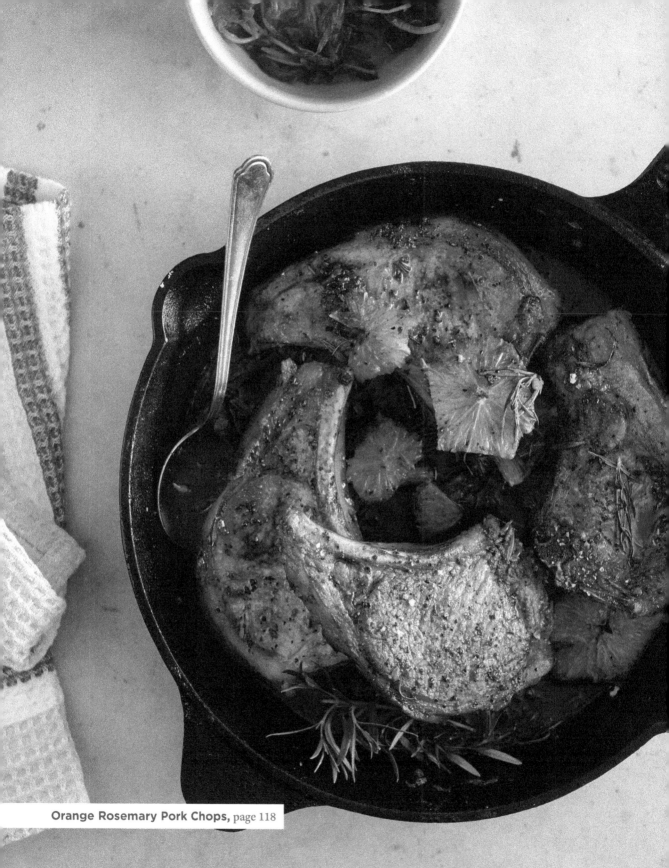

Orange Rosemary Pork Chops, page 118

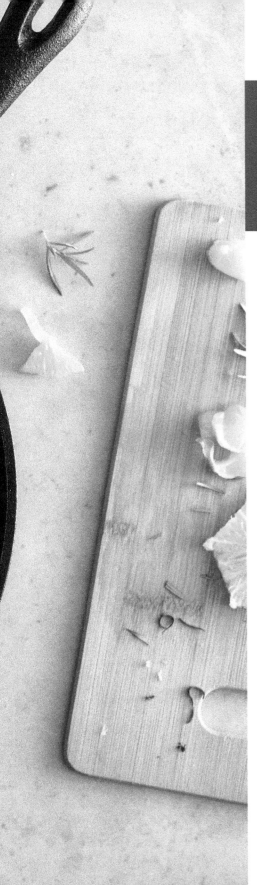

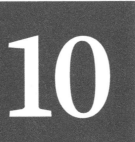

Beef, Pork, and Lamb

Spaghetti Squash with Savory Meat Sauce

Serves

6

PREP TIME:
10 MINUTES

COOK TIME:
1 HOUR
10 MINUTES

This delicious, savory meat sauce sneaks in some extra veggies and makes Italian food accessible without garlic cloves, which are high-FODMAP. You can also serve the sauce over any other tolerated type of gluten-free pasta or vegetable noodles. You also have the option of leaving the meat out of the sauce and substituting Sage Parmesan Meatballs (see page 110). If you want to use homemade sausage, see the recipe under Italian Sausage and Egg Scramble (page 58). If you are not doing a dairy-free diet, sprinkle some Parmesan cheese on top of this dish.

1 large spaghetti squash

¾ pound ground beef

¾ pound pork or homemade sausage

1 bunch scallions, chopped (green parts only)

1 tablespoon garlic-infused oil

1 small zucchini, peeled and chopped

1 red bell pepper, chopped

½ cup kalamata olives, drained and chopped

1 (26-ounce) carton strained tomatoes or tomato sauce (without garlic)

2 tablespoons Italian herbs (without garlic)

Sea salt

1. Preheat the oven to 425°F. Line a baking sheet with parchment paper or aluminum foil.

2. Pierce the spaghetti squash in several places with a sharp knife and place it on the baking sheet.

3. Bake the squash for about 40 minutes, or until a knife easily pierces the skin and there is little resistance in the flesh.

4. While the squash is baking, place the beef, pork, and scallions in a large skillet and cook over medium-high heat. Break up the meat into medium pieces with a spatula or wooden spoon. When the meat is cooked through, drain it if needed and set aside.

5. Heat the oil in a large saucepan or Dutch oven over medium heat.

6. Add the zucchini and bell pepper and sauté until they become tender, about 10 minutes.

7. Add the olives, tomatoes, Italian herbs, and ground meat mixture and stir to combine. Season with salt to taste. Simmer while preparing the squash. This will give the flavors time to meld.

8. Remove the squash from the oven and when it is cool enough to handle, halve it, remove the seeds, and scrape out the inside of the squash with a fork to create individual "spaghetti strands."

9. Divide the squash onto six plates and top each generously with meat sauce. Serve immediately.

▶ INGREDIENT TIP: Olives are recognized as a healthy food because they provide healthy fats that are connected to a positive decrease in cholesterol and blood pressure.

Per serving: Calories: 220; Total fat: 9g; Saturated fat: 2g; Cholesterol: 32mg; Sodium: 232mg; Carbohydrates: 18g; Fiber: 7g; Protein: 14g

Orange Rosemary Pork Chops

Serves

4

PREP TIME:
10 MINUTES

COOK TIME:
25 MINUTES

These pork chops are delicious and make a quick weeknight meal. The orange and rosemary really add an extra something to this dish, making it feel and taste like a special occasion. You can serve them with whatever vegetables you have handy, Sautéed Lemon Spinach (page 87), or Orange Carrot Purée (page 84).

2 oranges

4 bone-in, center-cut pork chops

1 tablespoon finely chopped fresh rosemary

Sea salt

Freshly ground black pepper

1 tablespoon ghee or avocado oil

1. Juice one orange and set the juice aside.

2. With a knife, remove the peel and pith from the second orange and cut the fruit into round slices. Set aside.

3. Pat each pork chop dry with a paper towel. Generously sprinkle the rosemary, salt, and pepper over both sides of each pork chop.

4. Heat a large skillet over medium-high heat and add the ghee to the pan once it is hot. When the ghee is heated, add the pork chops. Depending on the thickness of the pork chop, cook each side for 5 to 10 minutes, or until it is cooked through and a meat thermometer reaches 145°F.

5. Remove the pork chops and set each one on a plate. Add the reserved orange slices and juice to the pan. Cook for 1 to 2 minutes, stirring to scrape any brown bits from the pan. Pour the orange slices and juice over each plated pork chop. Serve immediately.

▶ **SIBO TIP:** For those on the Low-Histamine diet, do not use the oranges. Instead, add 1 tablespoon of unsalted butter, ghee, or garlic-infused oil when you would normally add the orange slices and juice to the pan to make the sauce at the end of the recipe.

Per serving: Calories: 215; Total fat: 9g; Saturated fat: 4g; Cholesterol: 67mg; Sodium: 50mg; Carbohydrates: 8g; Fiber: 2g; Protein: 25g

Steak with Tapenade Compound Butter

Serves

4

PREP TIME:
35 MINUTES

COOK TIME:
20 MINUTES

Going to a steakhouse is fun, but it is much more cost effective (and satisfying!) to make your own steak at home. It may feel daunting the first time you try it, but you will quickly learn how easy it is. When I had SIBO and low ferritin levels, I often craved red meat which made recipes like this perfect to make. While it's always a good idea to listen to what your cravings are telling you about your body, this steak recipe is a wonderful go-to for meat lovers.

4 tablespoons Tapenade Compound Butter (page 158)

1⅓ pounds boneless sirloin, rib eye, or comparable steak, or 4 individual bone-in steaks of ⅓ pound or more

2 tablespoons avocado oil or ghee

Sea salt

Freshly ground black pepper (optional)

1. Remove the compound butter from the refrigerator or freezer and divide it into four equal portions. Set aside and allow to come to room temperature.

2. Bring the steak to room temperature, about 30 minutes.

3. Pat both sides of the steak dry with paper towels.

4. Heat the oil in a large cast iron skillet over high heat.

5. Generously sprinkle both sides of the steak with salt and pepper (if using) to taste.

6. Add the steak to the pan and cook for 3 to 4 minutes for medium-rare doneness.

7. Flip the steak over and cook another 3 to 4 minutes.

8. Using a meat thermometer, check the temperature of the meat by inserting the thermometer through the thickest part of the steak and stopping in the middle; do not press the thermometer all the way down to the skillet. The temperature should register 135°F for medium rare, 145°F for medium, and 150°F for medium well.

9. Remove the steak from the skillet when it reaches your preferred temperature and let it rest for 5 minutes.

10. If you are cooking a single large steak, cut it against the grain and divide it among four serving plates. If you are cooking the four individual steaks, plate each one separately.

11. Top each steak with the compound butter. Serve immediately.

▶ INGREDIENT TIP: Always buy the best meat you can afford. Buying organic grass-fed meat from a local ranch or co-op is a great option, and it can be much more affordable to buy larger amounts of meat and freeze it.

Per serving: Calories: 557; Total fat: 47g; Saturated fat: 18g; Cholesterol: 112mg; Sodium: 422mg; Carbohydrates: 1g; Fiber: 0g; Protein: 31g

Shepherd's Pie

Serves

8

PREP TIME:
15 MINUTES

COOK TIME:
1 HOUR
5 MINUTES

Shepherd's pie originated in Ireland and has been around since the late 1700s. It was traditionally used as a way to turn leftovers into something new and delicious. On a SIBO diet, it makes a yummy main dish that incorporates a variety of flavors and that you can enjoy throughout the week.

FOR THE TOPPING

- 2 pounds medium white- or red-skinned potatoes
- 1 stick (8 tablespoons) salted butter or ghee
- ⅔ cup low-FODMAP milk, warmed
- Sea salt
- Freshly ground black pepper

FOR THE FILLING

- 1 tablespoon avocado oil or ghee
- 4 scallions, chopped (green parts only)
- 2 carrots, peeled and diced
- 1½ pounds ground beef or lamb
- 1 teaspoon sea salt
- ¼ teaspoon freshly ground black pepper
- 2 teaspoons Italian herbs (without garlic)
- 1 (14½-ounce) can fire-roasted tomatoes, drained (without garlic)
- Grated zest of 1 lemon

TO MAKE THE TOPPING

1. Peel the potatoes, place them in a medium saucepan, and cover them with water.

2. Bring the potatoes to a boil over high heat.

3. Reduce the heat to medium high and cook for about 20 minutes, or until the potatoes are soft and easily pierced with a fork.

4. Drain the potatoes and place them in a large bowl. Add the butter and milk and, using a mashing utensil or a hand mixer, blend the potatoes until smooth.

5. Season with salt and pepper to taste. Set aside.

TO MAKE THE FILLING

1. Preheat the oven to 400°F. Line a baking sheet with parchment paper or aluminum foil and set aside.

2. Place the oil in a large skillet and warm it over medium heat.

3. Add the scallions and carrots and sauté for 3 minutes, or until the vegetables begin to soften. Remove them from the skillet and set aside.

4. Place the ground beef, salt, pepper, and Italian herbs in a large skillet over medium heat and begin to break the meat into pieces with a spatula or wooden spoon.

5. Cook 10 to 12 minutes, or until the meat is browned. Remove from the heat, and drain any fat as needed.

6. Add the scallion-carrot mixture, tomatoes, and lemon zest to the meat mixture and stir to combine.

7. Transfer the mixture to a pie plate or a square 8-by-8-inch oven-safe pan.

8. Layer the mashed potatoes on top of the meat mixture.

9. Place the pie on the prepared baking sheet and bake in the oven for about 20 minutes, or until the top is lightly browned. Serve immediately.

▶ INGREDIENT TIP: If you do not tolerate potatoes, you can always substitute another puréed vegetable to top the pie. Puréed carrots or parsnips are good options.

Per serving: Calories: 352; Total fat: 19g; Saturated fat: 10g; Cholesterol: 85mg; Sodium: 507mg; Carbohydrates: 25g; Fiber: 3g; Protein: 20g

The Best Burgers

Makes
6
PATTIES

PREP TIME:
10 MINUTES

COOK TIME:
15 MINUTES

These burgers may contain basic ingredients, but the addition of pork sausage gives them a delicious taste. These are great to serve to a family of picky eaters since you can use regular buns or lettuce wraps and they are easily adaptable. Having a burger recipe is a wonderful thing for any cook, as you can customize your flavors with spices and even finely chopped vegetables for a different spin.

1 tablespoon Italian herbs (without garlic)

1 teaspoon sea salt, plus more to taste

1 tablespoon garlic-infused oil

1 pound ground beef

¾ pound ground pork

Freshly ground black pepper

1. In a large bowl, mix the Italian herbs, salt, oil, beef, and pork with your hands or a wooden spoon until thoroughly combined.

2. Shape the burgers into patties and sprinkle with salt and pepper to taste.

3. Cook for 5 to 7 minutes per side, or until the patties are cooked through.

▶ **MAKE-AHEAD TIP:** You can make a batch of burgers at the beginning of the week and take them for lunch a couple of times during the week, or freeze them in a storage bag for easy meals later. Use different toppings, such as cilantro chimichurri (see page 136), to give them a different taste.

Per serving (1 patty): Calories: 291; Total fat: 19g; Saturated fat: 7g; Cholesterol: 84mg; Sodium: 466mg; Carbohydrates: <1g; Fiber: <1g; Protein: 26g

Prosciutto-Wrapped Melon with Mint

Serves

4

PREP TIME:
15 MINUTES

You often see prosciutto and melon served as an appetizer, but I prefer it as a light summer meal. You can always add some soup on the side for something more substantial. If I am eating by myself, I will prepare the melon salad first and then wrap prosciutto around it as I go. If you are serving this as an appetizer, you can leave the melon salad and the prosciutto separate and supply toothpicks on the side so people can do it themselves. That way, they get to pick the portion size!

1 medium cantaloupe, cut into bite-size pieces

20 fresh mint leaves, julienned

¼ teaspoon freshly ground white pepper

3 tablespoons freshly squeezed lime juice

1 tablespoon olive oil

8 ounces prosciutto, halved

1. In a medium bowl, mix together the cantaloupe, mint, pepper, lime juice, and oil.

2. Wrap a half slice of prosciutto around one piece of dressed melon.

3. Spear a toothpick through the melon and prosciutto to keep it in place.

4. Repeat with the rest of the melon pieces. Serve immediately.

   ▶ SIBO TIP: If you are more of purist or if you are not sure what you are tolerating, eating just cantaloupe and prosciutto together is still quite a treat. Make sure that you buy good-quality prosciutto; its only ingredients should be pork and salt.

Per serving: Calories: 229; Total fat: 13g; Saturated fat: 5g; Cholesterol: 40mg; Sodium: 1,477mg; Carbohydrates: 15g; Fiber: 2g; Protein: 12g

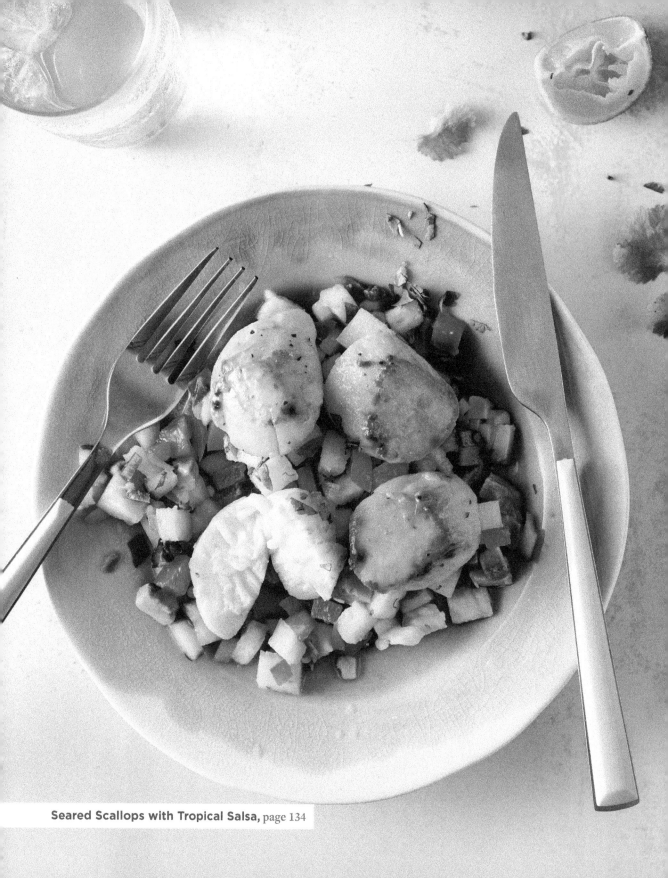

Seared Scallops with Tropical Salsa, page 134

11

Fish and Seafood

Easy Baked Salmon with Lemon and Thyme

Serves

4

***

PREP TIME:

10 MINUTES

***

COOK TIME:

20 MINUTES

This salmon recipe is great at the beginning of a SIBO diet because it is simple to make, and the omega-3 fatty acids in the fish have anti-inflammatory properties. It is also a light, healthy dish that goes well with rice or your preferred vegetables.

1 to 1½ pounds fresh salmon

Sea salt

Freshly ground black pepper

1 lemon, thinly sliced

2 tablespoons unsalted butter or ghee

2 thyme sprigs

1. Preheat the oven to 350°F. Line a baking sheet with parchment paper or aluminum foil.

2. Pat the salmon dry with a paper towel and generously season with salt and pepper on both sides. Set aside.

3. Lay half of the lemon slices on top of the parchment paper.

4. Place the salmon on top of the bed of lemon slices.

5. Dot the salmon with the butter and then top it with the other half of the lemon slices and the thyme.

6. Bake for 15 to 20 minutes, or until the fish is cooked through. Serve immediately.

▶ **SIBO TIP:** Farmed salmon tends to be cheaper than wild-caught salmon, but the latter has fewer pollutants, carcinogens linked to cancer, and antibiotic exposure. Long term, buying wild-caught salmon is money well spent.

Per serving: Calories: 167; Total fat: 8g; Saturated fat: 4g; Cholesterol: 70mg; Sodium: 137mg; Carbohydrates: 3g; Fiber: 1g; Protein: 23g

Pineapple Bacon Shrimp

Serves

2 to 4

PREP TIME:
15 MINUTES

COOK TIME:
35 MINUTES

I like to serve this as a main entrée because I am such a big fan of finger food. If you cannot find fresh pineapple, the canned version (only in pineapple juice, not syrup) will do the trick, or you can leave out the pineapple and just enjoy the bacon and shrimp solo. If you are buying shrimp by weight, large shrimp come to 33 shrimp per pound on average.

8 thick-cut bacon slices, halved

16 bite-size pieces of fresh pineapple

16 large raw shrimp, peeled, deveined, and tail removed

1 tablespoon avocado oil

¼ teaspoon sea salt

¼ teaspoon freshly ground white or black pepper

1. Preheat the oven to 400°F. Line two baking sheets with parchment paper or aluminum foil.

2. Place the bacon on one prepared baking sheet. Bake for about 15 minutes, turning once halfway through. The bacon should still be pliable and slightly more than halfway cooked. If you are using thinner bacon, cooking times will vary.

3. Remove the bacon from the oven and cool it on a wire rack until it is cool enough to touch, at least 5 minutes.

4. Place the shrimp in a small bowl and toss it with the oil, salt, and pepper.

5. Place one chunk of pineapple on top of one shrimp; then wrap one piece of bacon around the shrimp and pineapple and secure it with a toothpick. Place it on the second prepared baking sheet. Repeat with the rest of the shrimp.

CONTINUED ▶

6. Bake for 10 minutes, or until the shrimp are cooked and pink and the bacon is cooked through. Cool for 2 to 3 minutes, then serve.

▶ **INGREDIENT TIP:** There is much conflicting information as to whether bacon from healthy animals is okay to eat in moderation. The positive part is that it contains fat to keep you satiated and plenty of protein. My take on bacon is that people enjoy it wholeheartedly, both physically and emotionally, which has very positive aspects. So I say, unscientifically, to enjoy it thoroughly in moderation.

Per serving: Calories: 504; Total fat: 31g; Saturated fat: 9g; Cholesterol: 200mg; Sodium: 1,222mg; Carbohydrates: 11g; Fiber: 1g; Protein: 39g

Cod with Tomatoes and Pesto

Serves

4

PREP TIME:
10 MINUTES

COOK TIME:
15 MINUTES

Studies show that those who regularly eat fish tend to have lower risk of heart attack and heart disease. Cod is especially healthy because it is a good source of omega-3 fatty acids and vitamin B_6, as well as an excellent source of vitamin B_{12}, and people with SIBO often suffer from B_{12} deficiency. This method of cooking fish is called en papillote, a classic French cooking technique of steaming food in a parchment or aluminum foil packet, which allows the fish to soften and absorb wonderful flavors.

**4 fresh or defrosted
cod fillets**

1 teaspoon sea salt

**¼ teaspoon freshly
ground black pepper**

**¼ cup Fresh Basil
Pesto (page 157)**

**1 cup chopped tomatoes or
halved cherry tomatoes**

1. Preheat the oven to 400°F. Line a baking sheet with parchment paper or foil and then tear off four slightly smaller pieces of parchment paper.

2. Pat the cod dry with paper towels and season with salt and pepper.

3. Place each piece of cod on an individual piece of parchment paper.

4. Place 1 tablespoon of pesto on each fillet, spreading it out over the fillet.

5. Top the pesto with ¼ cup tomatoes.

6. Fold the sides of the parchment over the fish and then tuck the ends under to make a sealed package for each piece of fish.

CONTINUED ▶

7. Place the four cod packets on the prepared baking sheet and bake for 10 to 15 minutes, or until the fish flakes easily with a fork and is cooked through. Serve immediately.

▶ **INGREDIENT TIP:** You can substitute any type of mild white fish in this recipe, such as halibut or tilapia.

Per serving: Calories: 220; Total fat: 14g; Saturated fat: 2g; Cholesterol: 40mg; Sodium: 738mg; Carbohydrates: 2g; Fiber: <1g; Protein: 20g

Sardine Spread

Serves

2

PREP TIME:
**5 MINUTES,
PLUS 8 HOURS
TO CHILL**

This spread can serve as a light easy-to-make meal with some soup or bone broth. It can also be enjoyed with SIBO-friendly crackers or cucumber slices.

2 (4.4-ounce) tins wild sardines in water, drained

3 tablespoons unsalted butter or ghee (use ghee for CSD)

1 teaspoon freshly squeezed lemon juice

1 tablespoon olive oil

1 tablespoon garlic-infused oil

2 chopped scallions (green parts only)

2 tablespoons chopped fresh parsley

¼ teaspoon sea salt

¼ teaspoon freshly ground black pepper

1. Place the sardines, butter, lemon juice, olive oil, garlic-infused oil, scallions, parsley, salt, and pepper in a food processor and process until almost smooth.

2. Remove the spread from the food processor and put it in a small glass container. Refrigerate for 8 hours or overnight.

3. Allow the spread to come to room temperature before serving.

▶ **INGREDIENT TIP:** Sardines are high in protein and are a concentrated source of omega-3 fatty acids. They are also an excellent source of vitamins B_{12} and D, two vitamins that people with SIBO are often deficient in.

Per serving: Calories: 428; Total fat: 40g; Saturated fat: 16g; Cholesterol: 84mg; Sodium: 370mg; Carbohydrates: 1g; Fiber: 1g; Protein: 17g

Seared Scallops with Tropical Salsa

Serves

4

PREP TIME:
15 MINUTES

COOK TIME:
10 MINUTES

Other than a little bit of chopping, this is a very easy, healthy recipe—and a delicious one, which means more food diversity for you. If you know you tolerate spicy foods, add the jalapeño for a bit of heat. If you are unsure, err on the side of caution and leave it out; the recipe is packed with flavor either way. Use a small lime for this recipe, as a large one generally produces about 2 tablespoons of juice.

1⅓ **pounds dry scallops, tendons removed**

1 **cup finely chopped fresh pineapple**

½ **small avocado, pitted, peeled, and finely chopped**

½ **red bell pepper, finely chopped**

½ **cup finely chopped peeled and seeded cucumber**

3 **tablespoons chopped fresh cilantro**

½ **small jalapeño pepper, finely chopped (optional)**

¼ **teaspoon sea salt, plus more to taste**

Grated zest of 1 lime

1 **tablespoon freshly squeezed lime juice**

Freshly ground black pepper

2 **tablespoons avocado oil**

2 **tablespoons ghee or unsalted butter (use ghee for CSD)**

1. Pat the scallops dry with a paper towel and let them sit on a paper towel while you make the salsa.

2. To make the salsa, place the pineapple, avocado, bell pepper, cucumber, cilantro, jalapeño (if using), salt, lime zest, and lime juice in a medium bowl and mix well.

3. Pat the scallops again to make sure they are truly dry.

4. Sprinkle the scallops with salt and pepper to taste.

5. Heat a large sauté pan or skillet over high heat. Add the oil and let it heat until it is hot but not smoking.

6. Add the scallops in a single layer, flat-side down, leaving some space in between each one. It is okay to do the scallops in two batches as needed.

7. Cook the scallops for about 1½ minutes.

8. Add the ghee to the pan and then flip each scallop with tongs. Cook for another 1½ minutes while also spooning the melted ghee over the scallops to help them cook evenly.

9. Remove the scallops from the pan. Divide the salsa among each of four plates and place a quarter of the scallops on top of each. Serve immediately.

▶ INGREDIENT TIP: When you shop for scallops, make sure you go to a reputable fishmonger and ask for "dry" scallops. Dry scallops are those that have not been treated with sodium tripolyphosphate (STPP). Adding STPP preserves the scallops and helps them retain more water, making them weigh more and thus cost more. Dry scallops will get a nice sear from being cooked at high heat, whereas wet scallops tend to release water during the cooking process and therefore will not be able to get that nice crunchy outside.

Per serving: Calories: 335; Total fat: 21g; Saturated fat: 6g; Cholesterol: 39mg; Sodium: 148mg; Carbohydrates: 8g; Fiber: 2g; Protein: 14g

Baked Halibut with Cilantro Chimichurri

Serves

4

PREP TIME:
10 MINUTES

COOK TIME:
15 MINUTES

Halibut is such a versatile fish for an easy and quick but filling meal. Topping these flaky halibut fillets with fresh homemade cilantro chimichurri sauce adds incredible flavor to this dish. In this recipe, the chimichurri sauce really adds herbaceous flavor to the fish, and it is equally delicious when paired with sides such as roasted vegetables or potatoes.

1 pound halibut fillets

¼ teaspoon sea salt, plus more to taste

Freshly ground black pepper

2 bunches fresh cilantro

⅓ cup red wine vinegar

⅓ cup olive oil

¼ cup garlic-infused oil

1. Preheat the oven to 400°F. Line a baking sheet with parchment paper or aluminum foil.

2. Place the halibut fillets in the middle of the paper and generously season them with salt and pepper.

3. Bake for 15 minutes, or until the halibut is flaky.

4. While the halibut is cooking, make the chimichurri. Rinse and dry the cilantro, then cut off the top third of the bunch, where most of the leaves are. Discard the rest.

5. Place the cilantro, vinegar, olive oil, garlic-infused oil, and salt in a blender or food processor. Blend until puréed. Pour the chimichurri into a small bowl.

6. Divide the halibut between four serving plates and top each fillet generously with chimichurri. Serve immediately.

▶ **INGREDIENT TIP:** A chimichurri sauce traditionally uses parsley, but this version uses cilantro. Cilantro has antioxidant properties, and a 2011 study found that high doses of cilantro extract have anti-anxiety properties. If you do not care for cilantro, feel free to substitute parsley, which also has many health benefits.

Per serving: Calories: 418; Total fat: 35g; Saturated fat: 4g; Cholesterol: 45mg; Sodium: 229mg; Carbohydrates: 2g; Fiber: 1g; Protein: 24g

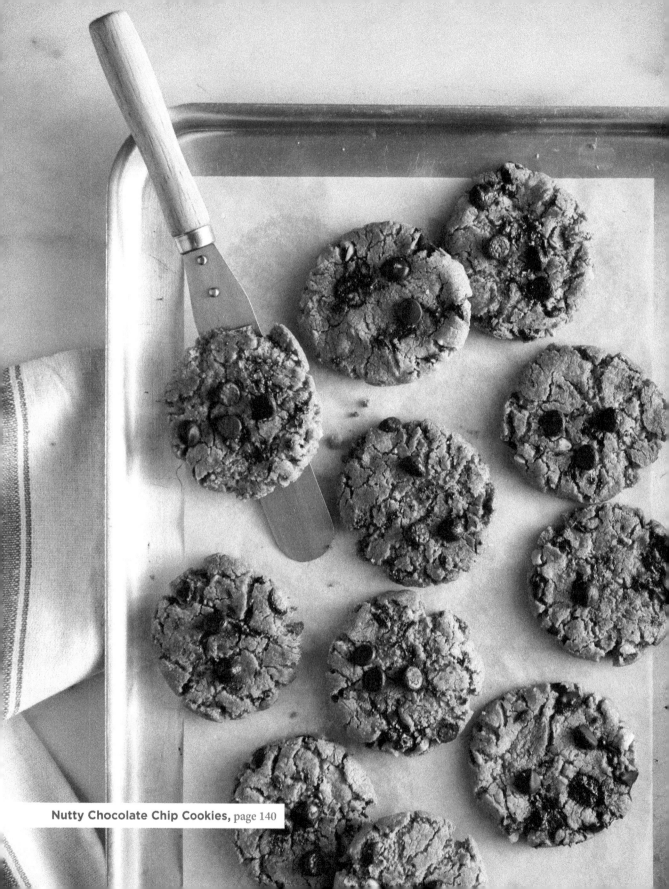

Nutty Chocolate Chip Cookies, page 140

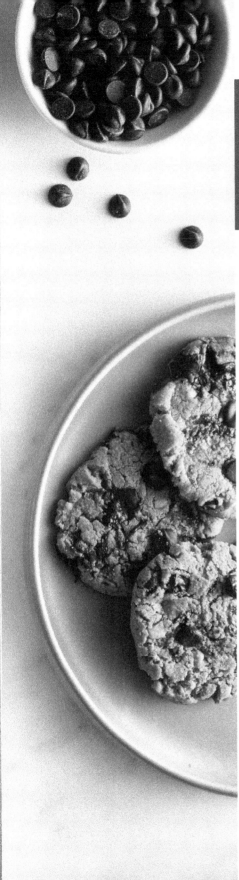

Desserts

Nutty Chocolate Chip Cookies

Makes
24
COOKIES

PREP TIME:
10 MINUTES

COOK TIME:
30 MINUTES

These nutty, delicious cookies are very simple, so they are easy to make on your own or with the whole family. They satisfy your sweet tooth but also give you a boost from healthy fats and protein in the almond butter. If you prefer regular chocolate chips, remember that this recipe will not be dairy-free.

½ teaspoon baking soda

¼ teaspoon kosher salt

¾ cup whole cane sugar

1 large egg, lightly beaten

¾ cup almond butter

¼ cup peanut butter

¾ cup dairy-free chocolate chips

1. Preheat the oven to 350°F. Line two baking sheets with silicone baking mats or parchment paper.

2. Put the baking soda, salt, and sugar in a large bowl and stir to mix.

3. Add the egg and mix. Then add the almond and peanut butters and mix until everything is thoroughly combined.

4. Add the chocolate chips and stir until evenly distributed.

5. Using your clean hands or a teaspoon, measure out teaspoon-size balls of cookie dough. Space the balls evenly on the prepared baking sheets, 12 per sheet.

6. Bake the cookies for 12 to 13 minutes.

7. Remove them from the oven, allow to cool on the baking sheet for 3 minutes, and then transfer them to a wire rack to cool further.

8. Store the cookies in a glass container at room temperature for up to one week.

▶ SIBO TIP: Make sure your chocolate chips are dairy-free. I also recommend buying dark chocolate, as it is better for you. But dark chocolate does contain fiber, so make sure you do not go overboard. Keep these cookies as a treat with only two per serving. You can also freeze and defrost them, or freeze the dough and defrost a portion when you want a freshly baked sweet treat.

Per serving (2 cookies): Calories: 248; Total fat: 17g; Saturated fat: 4g; Cholesterol: 15mg; Sodium: 135mg; Carbohydrates: 22g; Fiber: 3g; Protein: 5g

Double Chocolate Brownies

Makes
12
BROWNIES

PREP TIME:
10 MINUTES

COOK TIME:
25 MINUTES

Who doesn't love a brownie? This recipe is all about the deliciousness of chocolate, but, you can add less cocoa or fewer chocolate chips if you are sensitive to it. This is one of those recipes that will help you, and your family and friends, forget that you're eating a SIBO-centric diet. You'll just turn around and all the brownies will be gone. Maybe make a double batch?

1 teaspoon unsalted butter, ghee, or coconut oil (use ghee or coconut oil for CSD)

⅔ cup almond flour

¼ cup unsweetened cocoa powder

½ teaspoon ground cinnamon

½ teaspoon baking soda

⅔ cup whole cane sugar

⅛ teaspoon sea salt

½ cup olive oil

2 large eggs, beaten

2 teaspoons vanilla extract

¾ cup dairy-free chocolate chips or chopped dairy-free dark chocolate

1. Preheat the oven to 350°F. Grease an 8-by-8-inch square pan with the butter.

2. In a medium bowl, combine the flour, cocoa, cinnamon, baking soda, sugar, and salt. Mix thoroughly.

3. Make a well in the middle of the dry ingredients and add the oil, eggs, and vanilla. Mix thoroughly to combine with the dry ingredients.

4. Stir in the chocolate chips until just combined and evenly distributed.

5. Using a spatula, scrape the mixture into the prepared pan, smoothing the top to make it even. Bake for 25 minutes.

6. Remove the brownies from the oven and cool them on a wire rack. Cut and serve when cool.

▶ **INGREDIENT TIP:** Nuts can be hard to digest, so it is good to eat foods made with almond flour in smaller portions if you are not sure of your tolerance. The positive part about baking with almond flour is that almonds are high in monounsaturated fats—the same heart-healthy fat found in olive oil.

Per serving (1 brownie): Calories: 247; Total fat: 18g; Saturated fat: 5g; Cholesterol: 32mg; Sodium: 89mg; Carbohydrates: 19g; Fiber: 2g; Protein: 4g

GLUTEN-FREE • NUT-FREE • VEGETARIAN
DIETS: BPD (PHASE 2), CSD, LF, SCD, SSFG

Lemon Collagen Balls

Makes
20
BALLS

These lemon collagen balls are great to have around when you need a terrific dessert or snack. They are lemony, slightly sweet, and healthy, as they have added protein from the collagen and healthy fats from the coconut butter and oil.

PREP TIME:
15 MINUTES

½ cup coconut butter, softened

⅓ cup collagen

¼ cup almond flour

Grated zest of 1 lemon

3 tablespoons freshly squeezed lemon juice

1 tablespoon honey

1 tablespoon melted coconut oil

Shredded coconut, chopped nuts, or cocoa powder (optional), for coating

1. In a medium bowl, mix together the coconut butter, collagen, flour, lemon zest, lemon juice, honey, and oil until thoroughly combined.

2. Take a heaping teaspoon of the mixture and roll it into a ball. Roll each ball in the coconut (if using).

3. Continue until you have 20 balls or have used all the dough. Store in the refrigerator for up to one week.

▶ **SIBO TIP:** Some of my clients do great with coconut products, and some definitely do not. Before making this recipe, I would recommend eating a small amount (½ teaspoon or less) of coconut butter to test your tolerance.

Per serving (2 balls): Calories: 140; Total fat: 10g; Saturated fat: 8g; Cholesterol: 0mg; Sodium: 48mg; Carbohydrates: 5g; Fiber: 2g; Protein: 9g

Silky Olive Oil Custard

Serves

8

PREP TIME:
15 MINUTES

COOK TIME:
**35 MINUTES,
PLUS 1 HOUR
TO CHILL**

The addition of heart-healthy olive oil gives this custard an extra-creamy taste. This custard is great for the beginning of a SIBO diet because it is very simple to make. It also has few ingredients, making it much more likely to be tolerated. It combines protein from the eggs, carbohydrates from the honey or maple syrup, and healthy fat from the eggs and olive oil. You'll be coming back to this recipe time and time again because it is so delicious.

7 large eggs

½ cup honey or maple syrup (honey for BPD, SSFG, SCD and maple syrup for LF)

3 cups low-FODMAP milk

2 teaspoons vanilla extract

3 tablespoons olive oil

Pinch ground nutmeg

1. Preheat the oven to 350°F. Bring a kettle of water to a boil.

2. Put the eggs, honey, milk, vanilla, and oil in a blender and blend until well mixed, 1 to 2 minutes.

3. Pour the custard into eight individual ramekins or small bowls and set them on a roasting pan. Sprinkle nutmeg on top of each custard.

4. Pour the boiling water into the roasting pan so it reaches halfway up the sides of the ramekins. This creates a water bath for the custard.

5. Place the roasting pan in the oven and bake for 35 minutes. Remove the pan from the oven.

6. While wearing oven mitts, remove the individual ramekins from the hot water. Discard the hot water and place the ramekins in the refrigerator.

7. Chill the custard for at least 1 hour before serving.

▶ **COOKING TIP:** You can play around with the number of eggs to make the custard more or less "eggy," and with the cooking time to make the custard firmer or less solid. This method of baking with a tray of water is called a "water bath," and it adds moisture to the oven during the baking process. This is great for custards because they can become rubbery without moist heat in the oven.

Per serving: Calories: 205; Total fat: 11g; Saturated fat: 2g; Cholesterol: 163mg; Sodium: 95mg; Carbohydrates: 19g; Fiber: <1g; Protein: 8g

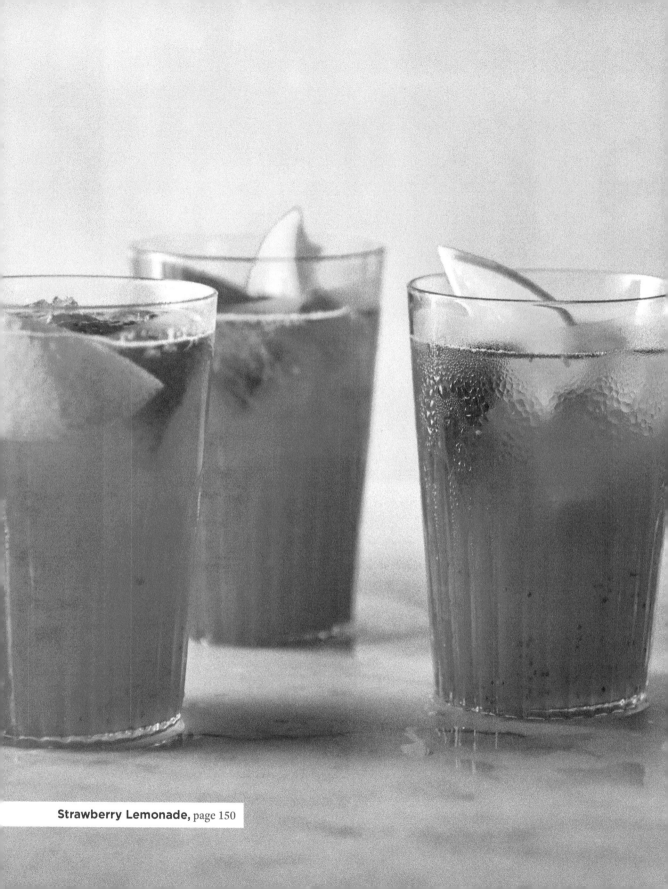

Strawberry Lemonade, page 150

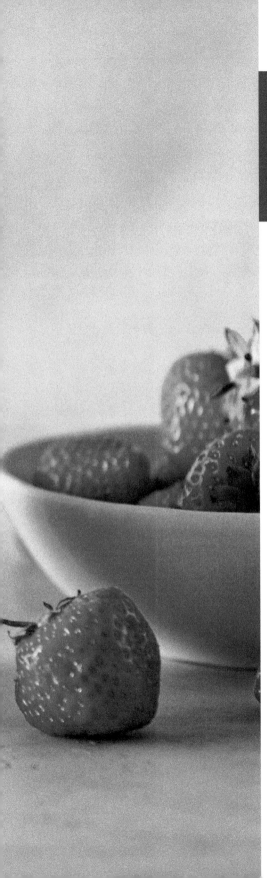

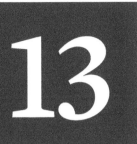

13

Drinks

149

DAIRY-FREE · GLUTEN-FREE · NUT-FREE · VEGETARIAN
DIETS: BPD (PHASE 1), CSD, LF, SCD, SSFG

Strawberry Lemonade

Serves

6

PREP TIME:
20 MINUTES

COOK TIME:
5 MINUTES

Adults and kids alike love this fruity lemonade. If you prefer an adult beverage with alcohol, vodka is SIBO-friendly and works well to create a fun summer cocktail. Just be judicious with the amounts; most people with SIBO tolerate only small amounts of alcohol. This recipe makes a simple syrup using water and honey or sugar as the sweet element.

¾ cup honey or whole cane sugar (use honey for SCD and SSFG and sugar for LF)

4¼ cups water, divided

2 cups fresh or defrosted frozen strawberries

1 cup freshly squeezed lemon juice

1. Put the honey and ¾ cup of water in a small saucepan over medium heat. Stir until well blended and fully liquid.

2. Remove from the heat, pour the simple syrup into a jar, and set the jar in the refrigerator to cool. Be careful about handling the jar, as the syrup will still be warm.

3. Using a hand mixer, blend the strawberries until they liquefy and no pieces remain.

4. Pour the strawberry purée, the remaining 3½ cups water, simple syrup, and lemon juice into a large pitcher. Stir until everything is mixed together.

5. Serve over ice. Store in the refrigerator for up to five days.

Per serving: Calories: 153; Total fat: 0g; Saturated fat: 0g; Cholesterol: 0mg; Sodium: 3mg; Carbohydrates: 42g; Fiber: 1g; Protein: 1g

DAIRY-FREE · GLUTEN-FREE · NUT-FREE · VEGETARIAN
DIETS: BPD (PHASE 1), CSD, LF, SCD, SSFG

Cucumber Mint Collagen Water

Serves

4

PREP TIME:
10 MINUTES

It is important to stay hydrated, and having tasty water around may inspire you to drink a bit more of it. You can add simple syrup (see the one used in the Strawberry Lemonade on page 150) to this cucumber mint water if you want a sweeter drink with more calories.

4 cups water

1 cucumber, peeled, seeded, and chopped

10 fresh mint leaves

¼ cup freshly squeezed lime juice

Grated zest of 2 limes

¼ cup collagen

1. Place the water, cucumber, mint, lime juice, and lime zest in a blender and process for about 1 minute, or until well blended.

2. Pour the mixture through a sieve or mesh strainer into a pitcher to remove any pulp.

3. Add the collagen to the pitcher and stir until it fully dissolves.

4. Serve immediately over ice or refrigerate for up to one week.

▶ **SIBO TIP:** Our body's production of collagen decreases as we age, so collagen supplementation can be very supportive. A 2003 study showed that collagen levels were decreased in patients with irritable bowel disease. The proline and glycine in collagen can also help repair damaged cell walls in the gut.

Per serving: Calories: 40; Total fat: 0g; Saturated fat: 0g; Cholesterol: 0mg; Sodium: 47mg; Carbohydrates: 3g; Fiber: 1g; Protein: 7g

Blueberry Milk

Serves

4

PREP TIME:
5 MINUTES

Blueberry milk sounds like something only kids would drink, but it is quite refreshing and a nice way to add calories through a beverage. I love this milk with breakfast. You can make it early in the week and store it in a pitcher or mason jar in the refrigerator for up to four days.

1 cup fresh or defrosted
   frozen blueberries

4 cups almond milk or
   other low-FODMAP milk

1 tablespoon honey or
   maple syrup (optional)

1 teaspoon vanilla
   extract (optional)

1. Place the blueberries, milk, honey (if using), and vanilla (if using) in a blender. Blend for 1 minute.

2. Strain the milk into a pitcher through a sieve or mesh strainer to remove any seeds or fruit pulp.

3. Serve immediately, or store for up to 4 days and stir it well before drinking.

▶ **SIBO TIP:** Any type of low-FODMAP berry can be used to make this milk. In this recipe, we use blueberries to ensure it is low-histamine.

Per serving: Calories: 65; Total fat: 2g; Saturated fat: 0g; Cholesterol: 0mg; Sodium: 160mg; Carbohydrates: 11g; Fiber: 2g; Protein: 1g

Maple Ginger Electrolyte Drink

Serves

4

PREP TIME:
15 MINUTES

COOK TIME:
10 MINUTES

Replacing electrolytes is important for everyone, but it becomes even more crucial if you are having diarrhea. Ginger can also reduce nausea and has potent anti-inflammatory effects.

3 cups water

1 (2-inch) knob fresh ginger, peeled and coarsely chopped

2 tablespoons maple syrup

¼ teaspoon sea salt

1 cup coconut water

¼ cup freshly squeezed lemon juice

1. Put the water, ginger, maple syrup, and salt in a medium saucepan over high heat.

2. Heat the mixture until just boiling, then remove from the heat and set aside to cool.

3. When the liquid is cool, remove the ginger by pouring the mixture through a sieve. Set the maple-ginger tea aside.

4. Add the coconut water and lemon juice to the maple-ginger tea in a pitcher or individual containers.

5. Serve it immediately over ice or refrigerate until cold.

▶ **SIBO TIP:** Coconut water is low-FODMAP in a 100-mL serving (slightly less than ½ cup). To keep this drink low-FODMAP, stick to a 1-cup serving of the electrolyte drink per meal.

Per serving: Calories: 45; Total fat: 0g; Saturated fat: 0g; Cholesterol: 0mg; Sodium: 153mg; Carbohydrates: 12g; Fiber: 0g; Protein: 0g

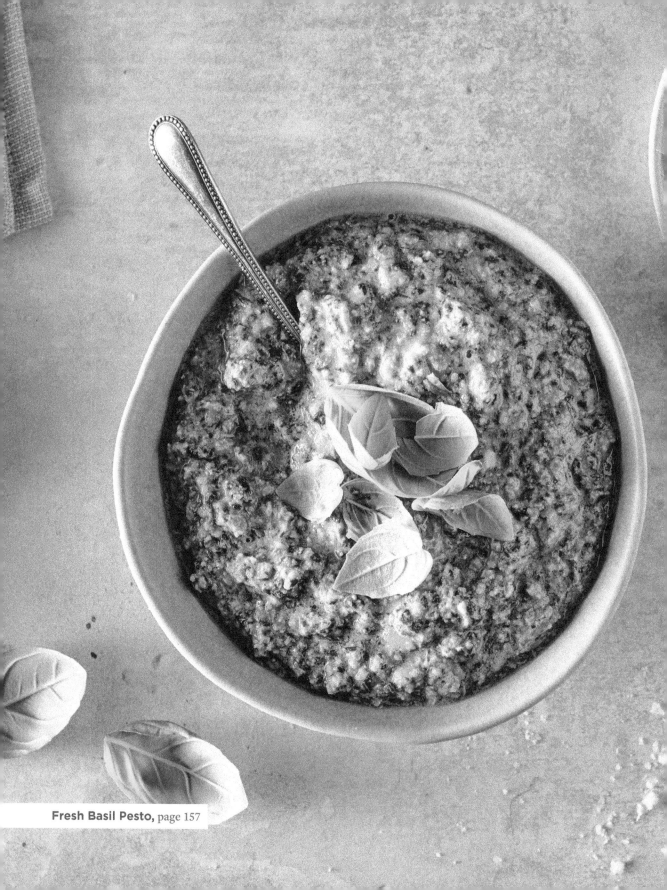

Fresh Basil Pesto, page 157

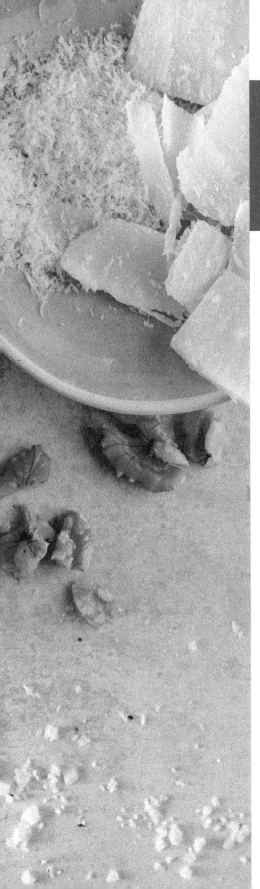

14

Sauces, Condiments, and Dressings

GLUTEN-FREE • NUT-FREE • VEGETARIAN
DIETS: BPD (PHASE 1), CSD, LF, SCD, SSFG

Zesty Hollandaise Sauce

Serves

8

PREP TIME:
5 MINUTES

COOK TIME:
5 MINUTES

Hollandaise sauce is rich, so a little goes a long way. It tastes amazing over steak, eggs, or vegetables like broccoli. Even though it is quite easy to make, it is impressive to make when having company over for a meal, and it's incredibly delicious.

4 egg yolks

2 tablespoons freshly squeezed lemon juice

Pinch of freshly ground black pepper (optional)

½ cup salted butter or ghee (use ghee for CSD)

2 tablespoons water

1. Put the egg yolks, lemon juice, and pepper (if using) in a blender. Set aside.

2. Put the butter and water in a small saucepan over medium heat. Stir them together while the butter melts and then bubbles.

3. Start the blender and then quickly remove the middle portion of the blender cover.

4. Pour the butter-water mixture in a slow stream into the blender while the blender continues to run.

5. The sauce will begin to thicken as you add the butter-water mixture. It should take 30 to 60 seconds total. Once sauce is thickened, serve immediately.

▶ **COOKING TIP:** It is important to serve hollandaise sauce immediately; otherwise, it will begin to congeal. To help prevent congealing, put the sauce in a small bowl set in warm water.

Per serving: Calories: 130; Total fat: 14g; Saturated fat: 8g; Cholesterol: 123mg; Sodium: 86mg; Carbohydrates: <1g; Fiber: 0g; Protein: 1g

Fresh Basil Pesto

Serves

4

PREP TIME:
10 MINUTES

This pesto is quite easy to make, especially during the summer months when basil is plentiful. However, if you don't have access to fresh basil or want to make pesto in another season, you can always substitute spinach, arugula, or other greens for the basil in this easy but flavor-packed sauce.

¼ **cup olive oil**

¼ **cup garlic-infused oil**

1 cup packed fresh basil leaves

2 teaspoons freshly squeezed lemon juice

¼ **cup chopped walnuts or almonds (optional)**

¼ **cup freshly shredded Parmesan cheese (optional)**

¼ **teaspoon sea salt**

1. Put the olive oil, garlic-infused oil, basil, lemon juice, walnuts (if using), Parmesan (if using), and salt in a food processor. Blend until all the ingredients are puréed, stopping to scrape down the sides of the blender as needed.

2. Serve the pesto immediately, or transfer it to a food storage container and refrigerate for up to 1 week.

▶ **SIBO TIP:** If you want this pesto to be nut-free or dairy-free, leave out the nuts or the cheese. I typically make it without dairy, and as long as I add enough salt, I really cannot taste the difference.

Per serving: Calories: 241; Total fat: 27g; Saturated fat: 4g; Cholesterol: 0mg; Sodium: 146mg; Carbohydrates: <1g; Fiber: <1g; Protein: <1g

Tapenade Compound Butter

Serves

8

PREP TIME:

15 MINUTES

This tapenade compound butter is great to make in advance and store in the refrigerator like regular butter, or freeze it for later use. Simply cut off a slice and place it on top of hot, cooked chicken, pork, beef, or roasted vegetables to add delicious, buttery flavor.

1 (6-ounce) jar pitted kalamata olives, drained

½ teaspoon anchovy paste

1 tablespoon drained capers

½ teaspoon Italian herbs (without garlic)

1 tablespoon garlic-infused oil

1 stick unsalted butter, softened

1. Put the olives, anchovy paste, capers, herbs, and oil in a food processor or blender and blend until well mixed and still slightly chunky.

2. Transfer the tapenade to a medium bowl. Add the butter and mix it thoroughly into the tapenade.

3. Place the tapenade butter on a piece of parchment paper or aluminum foil and fold the paper over it to make a log form. Tuck the remaining parchment under and seal the edges with tape if needed.

4. Store the tapenade compound butter in the refrigerator.

▶ **INGREDIENT TIP:** You can experiment with adding citrus juice, zest, fresh herbs, honey, or spices to get diverse flavors.

Per serving: Calories: 173; Total fat: 19g; Saturated fat: 8g; Cholesterol: 32mg; Sodium: 342mg; Carbohydrates: 1g; Fiber: <1g; Protein: <1g

GLUTEN-FREE • NUT-FREE • VEGETARIAN
DIETS: BPD (PHASE 2), LF, SCD, SSFG

Ranch Dressing

Serves

4

PREP TIME:
10 MINUTES

The key ingredient in this ranch dressing recipe, 24-hour yogurt, is a major staple for a SIBO diet. You can use this ranch dressing as a soup topping instead of sour cream, or as a dip for chicken wings. You may find many ways to use yogurt in SIBO recipes, but this ranch dressing is one of my favorites.

1 cup 24-Hour Yogurt (page 64) or store-bought lactose-free yogurt

1 tablespoon garlic-infused oil

⅓ cup shredded Parmesan cheese

¼ teaspoon paprika

1 tablespoon chopped fresh chives

1 tablespoon chopped fresh parsley

½ teaspoon sea salt

¼ teaspoon freshly ground black pepper

1. Place all the ingredients in a small bowl and mix thoroughly.

2. Taste and add more salt as needed (enough salt changes the yogurt from tasting like yogurt to more like ranch dressing).

3. Refrigerate in a glass storage container for up to 1 week.

▶ **INGREDIENT TIP:** The 24-Hour Yogurt has a high probiotic load because of the 24-hour fermentation time. Probiotic yogurts have been found to decrease overall blood cholesterol levels while increasing HDL cholesterol. Yogurt is also helpful in regulating blood sugar.

Per serving: Calories: 107; Total fat: 8g; Saturated fat: 3g; Cholesterol: 14mg; Sodium: 475mg; Carbohydrates: 4g; Fiber: 0g; Protein: 5g

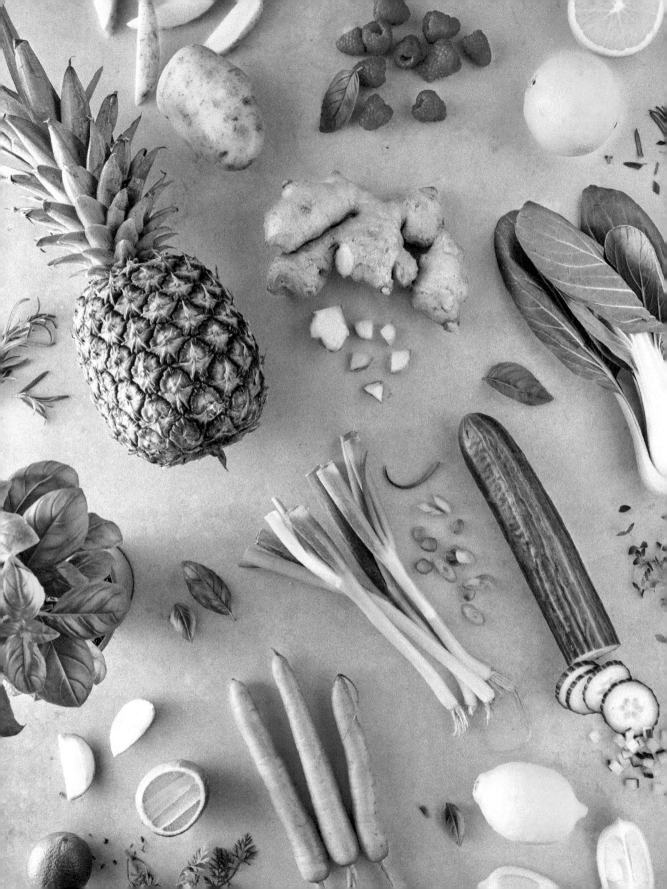

The Low-FODMAP Dirty Dozen™

These lists are adapted from the Environmental Working Group's (ewg. org) Dirty Dozen™ and Clean Fifteen™ lists, tailored to include only low-FODMAP fruits and vegetables. NOTE: Some of these are high FODMAP in specific amounts, so be sure to check.

The Dirty Dozen™ are the fruits and vegetables best purchased as organic because, if conventionally grown, they contain a lot of pesticides. This list is in order of most to least contaminated:

DIRTY DOZEN™

1. Strawberries
2. Spinach
3. Grapes
4. Celery
5. Tomatoes
6. Sweet bell peppers
7. Potatoes
8. Cucumbers
9. Cherry tomatoes
10. Lettuce
11. Blueberries, domestic
12. Kale and collard greens

The Low-FODMAP Clean Seven

This list has been reduced to seven low-FODMAP fruits and vegetables that are relatively low in pesticides. These are safe to buy as conventionally grown and are listed starting with the least contaminated in the group. NOTE: Some of these are high FODMAP in specific amounts, so be sure to check.

CLEAN SEVEN

1. Avocado
2. Pineapple
3. Cabbage
4. Eggplant
5. Honeydew melon
6. Kiwi
7. Cantaloupe

Measurement Conversions

VOLUME EQUIVALENTS (LIQUID)

STANDARD	US STANDARD (OUNCES)	METRIC (APPROXIMATE)
2 tablespoons	1 fl. oz.	30 mL
¼ cup	2 fl. oz.	60 mL
½ cup	4 fl. oz.	120 mL
1 cup	8 fl. oz.	240 mL
1½ cups	12 fl. oz.	355 mL
2 cups or 1 pint	16 fl. oz.	475 mL
4 cups or 1 quart	32 fl. oz.	1 L
1 gallon	128 fl. oz.	4 L

OVEN TEMPERATURES

FAHRENHEIT (F)	CELSIUS (C) (APPROXIMATE)
250°	120°
300°	150°
325°	165°
350°	180°
375°	190°
400°	200°
425°	220°
450°	230°

VOLUME EQUIVALENTS (DRY)

STANDARD	METRIC (APPROXIMATE)
⅛ teaspoon	0.5 mL
¼ teaspoon	1 mL
½ teaspoon	2 mL
¾ teaspoon	4 mL
1 teaspoon	5 mL
1 tablespoon	15 mL
¼ cup	59 mL
⅓ cup	79 mL
½ cup	118 mL
⅔ cup	156 mL
¾ cup	177 mL
1 cup	235 mL
2 cups or 1 pint	475 mL
3 cups	700 mL
4 cups or 1 quart	1 L

WEIGHT EQUIVALENTS

STANDARD	METRIC (APPROXIMATE)
½ ounce	15 g
1 ounce	30 g
2 ounces	60 g
4 ounces	115 g
8 ounces	225 g
12 ounces	340 g
16 ounces or 1 pound	455 g

Resources

WEBSITES

Bristol Stool Scale: https://en.wikipedia.org/wiki/Bristol_stool_scale
A general scale for quality bowel movements.

Clean Fifteen™: www.ewg.org/foodnews/clean-fifteen.php

Environmental Working Group: www.ewg.org
Source for the annual Dirty Dozen™ and Clean Fifteen™ lists, their guides to the fruits and vegetables with the most and least amount of pesticides.

Dirty Dozen™: www.ewg.org/foodnews/dirty_dozen_list.php# .WlOV8FQ-dTY

Gemelli Biotech: www.gemellibiotech.com/products
This offers IBS blood tests and a possible upcoming hydrogen-sulfide breath test.

Monash University Low-FODMAP Diet app: www.monashfodmap .com/i-have-ibs/get-the-app/
This app offers the most up-to-date and scientifically tested FODMAP list available.

QuinTron SIBO Lactulose and Glucose Testing: www.breathtests.com

SIBO–Small Intestine Bacterial Overgrowth: www.siboinfo.com
Dr. Allison Siebecker's website is a wealth of free information about SIBO.

SIBO SOS: https://sibosos.com/
Summits, podcasts, online courses, and resources.

Vital Food Therapeutics: www.vitalfoodtherapeutics.com
Kristy Regan's site offers free SIBO-friendly recipes and information.

The World's Healthiest Foods: www.whfoods.com/foodstoc.php
This website offers free scientifically based information on the healthiest foods.

DIET INFORMATION

Histamine Intolerance
Dr. Nirala Jacobi's SIBO/Histamine SIBO/Bi-Phasic Diet:
www.thesibodoctor.com/sibo-histamine-bi-phasic-diet-download/

Histamine Intolerance Awareness: https://www.histamineintolerance
.org.uk/about/the-food-diary/the-food-list/

Hydrogen Sulfide SIBO and Low-Sulfur Diets
Discussion with dietitian Heidi Turner: https://drruscio.com
/diets-sulfur-intolerance-with-heidi-turner/

Discussion with Dr. Greg Nigh: www.thesibodoctor.com/2017/12/20
/sibo-and-hydrogen-sulfide/?v=7516fd43adaa

Discussion with Dr. Nirala Jacobi: https://drruscio.com
/hydrogen-sulfide-sibo-treatment/

Living Network's High- and Low-Sulfur (Thiols) Foods List:
http://www.livingnetwork.co.za/chelationnetwork/food
/high-sulfur-sulphur-food-list/

FOODS & PRODUCTS

Casa de Sante low-FODMAP soup, stock, and broth:
https://casadesante.com/collections/certified-low-fodmap
-soup-broth

Castor oil packs: available on Amazon.

Collagen hydrolysate: Great Lakes Collagen Hydrolysate or Vital
Proteins Collagen Peptides, both available on Amazon.

Gut Rx Gurus Low-FODMAP Bone Broth: https://gutrxbonebroth.com/

Integrative Therapeutics Elemental Diet: www.integrativepro.com
/Products/Gastrointestinal/Physicians-Elemental-Diet-Dextrose-Free

Low-FODMAP prepared foods: www.fodyfoods.com/collections/all

WORKSHOPS, RETREATS, AND CONFERENCES

Russell Delman: www.russelldelman.com
Workshops and retreats for developing presence and gratitude.

SIBO Con 2020: www.synergycmegroup.com/2020-integrative
-sibo-confe
This is a clinical-focused SIBO conference.

**SIBO Symposium at National University of Natural Medicine (NUNM)
for both doctors and patients:**
https://career-alumni.nunm.edu/continuing-education/2019-sibo
-symposium

References

Bowe, Whitney P., and Alan C. Logan. "Acne Vulgaris, Probiotics and the Gut-Brain-Skin Axis—Back to the Future?" *Gut Pathogens* 3, no. 1 (January 2011): 1. doi:10.1186/1757-4749-3-1.

Chedid, Victor, Sameer Dhalla, John O. Clarke, Bani Chander Roland, Kerry B. Dunbar, Joyce Koh, Edmundo Justino, et al. "Herbal Therapy Is Equivalent to Rifaximin for the Treatment of Small Intestinal Bacterial Overgrowth." *Global Advances in Health and Medicine* 3, no. 3 (May 2014): 16–24. doi:10.7453/gahmj.2014.019.

Environmental Working Group. "Arsenic Is in Rice—Should You Worry?" Accessed July 15, 2019. https://www.ewg.org/foodscores/content/arsenic-contamination-in-rice.

Foran, Jeffery A., David H. Good, David O. Carpenter, M. Coreen Hamilton, Barbara A. Knuth, and Steven J. Schwager. "Quantitative Analysis of the Benefits and Risks of Consuming Farmed and Wild Salmon." *Journal of Nutrition* 135, no. 11 (November 2005): 2639–43. doi:10.1093/jn/135.11.2639.

Fujimori, Shunji. "What Are the Effects of Proton Pump Inhibitors on the Small Intestine?" *World Journal of Gastroenterology* 21, no. 22 (June 2015): 6817-19. doi.org/10.3748/wjg.v21.i22.6817.

Huang, Ting-Ting, Jian-Bo Lai, Yan-Li Du,Yi Xu, Lie-Min Ruan, and Shao-Hua Hu. "Current Understanding of Gut Microbiota in Mood Disorders: An Update of Human Studies." *Frontiers in Genetics* 10, no. 98 (February 2019). doi:10.3389/fgene.2019.00098.

International Foundation for Functional Gastrointestinal Disorders. "Facts about IBS." Last modified November 24, 2016. https://www.aboutibs.org/facts-about-ibs.html.

Kelesidis, Theodoros, and Charalabos Pothoulakis. "Efficacy and Safety of the Probiotic *Saccharomyces boulardii* for the Prevention and Therapy of Gastrointestinal Disorders." *Therapeutic Advances in Gastroenterology* 5, no. 2 (March 2012): 111–25. doi:10.1177/1756283X11428502.

Koutroubakis, Ioannis, Efi Petinaki, Philippos Dimoulios, Emmanouel Vardas, Maria Roussomoustakaki, Antonios N. Maniatis, and Elias Kouroumalis. "Serum Laminin and Collagen IV in Inflammatory Bowel Disease." *Journal of Clinical Pathology* 56, no. 11 (November 2003): 817–20. doi:10.1136/jcp.56.11.817.

Luo, Yuanyuan, Benhua Zeng, Li Zeng, Xiangyu Du, Bo Li, Ran Huo, Lanxiang Liu, et al. "Gut Microbiota Regulates Mouse Behaviors through Glucocorticoid Receptor Pathway Genes in the Hippocampus." *Translational Psychiatry* 8, no. 187 (September 2018): 187. doi:10.1038/s41398-018-0240-5.

Mahendra, Poonam, and Shradha Bisht. "Anti-Anxiety Activity of *Coriandrum sativum* Assessed Using Different Experimental Anxiety Models." *Indian Journal of Pharmacology* 43, no. 5 (September 2011): 574–77. doi:10.4103/0253-7613.84975.

Nehra, Avinash K., Jeffrey A. Alexander, Conor G. Loftus, and Vandana Nehra. "Proton Pump Inhibitors: Review of Emerging Concerns." *Mayo Clinic Proceedings* 93, no. 2 (February 2018): 240–46. doi.org/10.1016/j.mayocp.2017.10.022.

Parodi, Andrea, Stefania Paolino, Alfredo Greco, Francesco Drago, Carlo Mansi, Alfredo Rebora, Aurora Parodi, and Vincenzo Savarino. "Small Intestinal Bacterial Overgrowth in Rosacea: Clinical Effectiveness of Its Eradication." *Clinical Gastroenterology and Hepatology* 6, no. 7 (July 2008): 759–64. doi.org/10.1016/j.cgh.2008.02.054.

Pimentel, Mark, Evelyn Chow, and Henry Lin. "Normalization of Lactulose Breath Testing Correlates with Symptom Improvement in Irritable Bowel Syndrome: A Double-Blind, Randomized, Placebo-Controlled Study." *American Journal of Gastroenterology* 98, no. 2 (February 2003): 412–19. doi.org/10.1016/S0002-9270(02)05902-6.

Pimentel, Mark, Tess Constantino, Yuthana Kong, Meera Bajwa, Abolghasem Rezaei, and Sandy Park. "A 14-Day Elemental Diet Is Highly Effective in Normalizing the Lactulose Breath Test." *Digestive Diseases and Sciences* 49, no. 1 (January 2004): 73–7. doi.org/10.1023/B:DDAS.0000011605.43979.e1.

Rey, Frederico E., Mark D. Gonzalez, Jiye Cheng, Meng Wu, Philip P. Ahern, and Jeffrey I. Gordon. "Metabolic Niche of a Prominent Sulfate-Reducing Human Gut Bacterium." *Proceedings of the National Academy of Sciences* 110, no. 33 (August 2013): 13582–87. doi.org/10.1073/pnas.1312524110.

Rezaie A, Michelle C. Buresi, Anthony Lembo, and Henry Lin. "Hydrogen and Methane-Based Breath Testing in Gastrointestinal Disorders: The North American Consensus." *The American Journal of Gastroenterology* 112, no. 5 (March 2017): 775–84. doi:10.1038/ajg.2017.46.

Index

Acknowledgments

TO THOSE LIVING WITH SIBO, please know that this healing journey will contain both challenging hardships and great gifts. Gratitude and wholeness are within reach. I am honored to be a part of your journey.

Thank you to my dear husband, Gregg. It means the world to me to always have you by my side through thick and thin.

My gratitude to my clients, who continue to remind me why I do this work.

Many thanks to Dr. Sandberg-Lewis for contributing the foreword as well as for his continued support and mentorship.

I am so grateful to be part of a community of dedicated health-care providers. Thank you for your generosity, support, humor, and intelligence. In particular, my gratitude goes to Dr. Allison Siebecker, Shivan Sarna, Dr. Lisa Shaver, Dr. Megan Taylor, Dr. Crane Holmes, Dr. Julie Briley, Dr. Pera Gorson, Julie Marks, Dr. Roz Donovan, Heidi Turner, Dr. Louise Rose, and Rebecca Coomes.

Thank you to my Monthly Accountability Group friends and colleagues Marne Bishop and Karen Davis. You are always inspiring and supportive.

There are too many dear friends to thank them all here, but during this time, I am especially grateful to Mary Gelinas, Jenn Fieldhack, Jodi Friedman, Andrea Richards, Kristin Furuichi, Kristina Sacks, and Nichole Alvarado.

Thank you to my parents, siblings (extra kudos to Dan for buying my last book and sending me a picture with it!), sibling-in-laws (I really consider you siblings), niece, nephews, aunts, uncles, and cousins. I love traveling through life with you.

About the Author

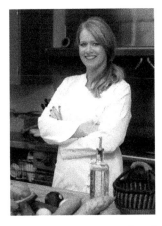

KRISTY REGAN is a holistic nutritionist specializing in gastrointestinal disorders. She studied at National University of Natural Medicine, where she earned her master of science in nutrition. Her practice combines nutritional therapy, lifestyle education, and counseling to assist clients in their healing journeys. She appreciates how important it is to connect and address both physical and emotional health. After her own multiyear journey with SIBO, she is proud to say it is possible to heal.

Kristy co-organized and spoke at the 2019 NUNM SIBO Symposium. She has been featured on three online SIBO summits, wrote the book *The SIBO Diet Plan*, and has a SIBO Soothe and Manage program available on the Suggestic app.

She is passionate about sharing her insights and expertise in cooking, nutrition, health, and mind-body therapies via podcasts, classes, and speaking engagements. Kristy is available for individual nutrition and wellness appointments online worldwide. Visit her website, VitalFoodTherapeutics.com, for free recipes and digestive health information.

Printed in the USA
CPSIA information can be obtained
at www.ICGtesting.com
LVHW052135091223
765798LV00002B/23

9 781641 529860